STRAIGHT TALK

about

BREAST CANCER

FROM DIAGNOSIS TO RECOVERY

SUZANNE W. BRADDOCK, M.D.
JANE M. KERCHER, M.D.
JOHN J. EDNEY, M.D.
MELANIE MORRISSEY CLARK

616.99
S

Addicus Books
Omaha, Nebraska

An Addicus Nonfiction Book

ISBN# 1-886039-60-7
Cover design by Peri Paloni
Illustrations by Jack Kusler
Photos by Larry S. Ferguson and Paula Friedland

This book is not intended to serve as a substitute for a physician. Nor is it the authors' intent to give medical advice contrary to that of an attending physician.

Library of Congress Cataloging-in-Publication Data

Straight talk about breast cancer from diagnosis to recovery / Suzanne W. Braddock ... [et al.].
    p. cm.
  Includes index.
  ISBN 1-886039-60-7 (alk. paper)
  1. Breast—Cancer—Popular works. I. Braddock, Suzanne W., 1942-
RC280.b8 S748 2002
616.99'449—dc21   2002003218

Addicus Books, Inc.
P.O. Box 45327
Omaha, Nebraska 68145
Web site: http://www.AddicusBooks.com

Printed in the United States of America
10 9 8 7 6 5 4 3 2 1

To all women diagnosed with breast cancer and their families.

Contents

Preface

Please read this book imagining that a very good friend is sitting close to you, giving you this introduction to the rest of your life with love and understanding. Imagine your friend—who has indeed walked in your shoes—taking you by the hand and guiding you through the next few weeks.

Your friend wants to help you understand what is happening, and help you cope with the decisions and treatments ahead. She also wants to help your family and friends, for they are suffering with you.

Know there will come a time when you will go entire minutes without thinking of breast cancer—then hours, and even days. Of course, your life will never be the same. In fact, it will most likely be better in many ways you would not have chosen, but will be delighted to discover.

The authors of this book reach out to you as dear friends and offer you the hope of a complete recovery, along with the certainty that the journey from here will be one of growth, challenge, and change. That is, after all, what life is about.

Acknowledgments

We would like to thank the many individuals who shared their time and expertise so generously to help make this book possible. We thank several physicians for their contributions to the book's content. They include: Dr. Margaret Block, Dr. Bob Langdon Jr., Dr. Patrick J. McKenna, Dr. Janalyn Prows, Dr. Henry Lynch, Dr. Ramon Fusaro, Dr. John J. Heieck, Dr. Richard J. Bruneteau, Dr. Paul Ruggieri, and Rosalind Benedet, NP, MSN.

We acknowledge Mollie Foster, Ph.D., for her contributions to the coping chapter and Judy Dierkhising, Ph.D., for her input on dealing with the emotional needs of breast cancer patients. We also are grateful to members of the Nebraska Methodist Hospital Breast Cancer Support Group for their comments, wit, and strength. And with gratitude, we remember the late Sue Kocsis, a real spark, whose encouragement meant so much during the early stages of this book.

The authors also are deeply grateful to the women who answered personal and sometimes painful questions in order to help others. Their comments taught us how strength and hope can triumph over despair.

To the women who shared their surgery and reconstruction in photographs, a very special thank-you. We also acknowledge photographers Larry Ferguson and Paula Friedland for their creativity and sensitivity in portraying these women not as medical results but as real, living women. We thank Kate Maloy for her expert editorial support and Jack Kusler for the illustrations he provided for the book.

Introduction

Someone you love or someone you know will get breast cancer. Your friend, your aunt, your mother, your daughter, yourself. The fact is, if you are an American woman, your risk is especially high. If we all live to age eighty-five, 1 in 8 women in the United States will have suffered breast cancer. Each year, on average, it strikes about 180,000 women. But the good news is, more and more women with breast cancer are surviving. And not just five-year, disease-free survival, either. Real, long-lasting, bounce-the-grandkids-on-your-knee survival.

My Journey Through Breast Cancer

The rest of my life started April 1, 1992, with a phone call from my friend and doctor, who informed me that a lump in my breast had been diagnosed malignant. I reacted, as do most women, with the irrational certainty that I was going to die, and soon. I was forty-nine.

Although I am a physician—a dermatologist—I knew little more about breast cancer than I had learned in medical school in the late 1970s. Back then, I saw several patients who died from the disease, and I was afraid. So I dutifully saw my physician every year for an exam (right), had a baseline mammogram between ages thirty-five and forty (right), and had a mammogram every other year between forty and fifty (right). I also began planning for annual mammograms when I was about to turn fifty (right—though experts now recommend annual mammograms after age forty). I also practiced breast self-examinations on a "regularly sporadic" basis (wrong). Like many women, I had "lumpy" breasts, making self-examination difficult to interpret. I relied on my physicians and mammograms to keep me safe (very wrong).

I was disappointed that three doctors examined me many times and failed to recommend a biopsy—a test that takes a tissue sample and analyzes it for cancer. I was disheartened that mammograms failed to detect my cancer. But I was most amazed that I had been so cavalier with the very things that could have diagnosed my tumor sooner: regular, monthly breast self-exams and insistence on having a biopsy done on a lump that worried me. Denial is a powerful thing.

Fortunately, my cancer had not yet spread when it was diagnosed, at least as far as current technology could determine. The tumor was medium-sized—2.2 centimeters, a little less than one inch.

Surgery is almost always recommended for breast cancer. I chose to have a mastectomy. Then, like many other breast cancer patients, I underwent chemotherapy. Women with breast cancer are offered chemotherapy when their tumors are of a certain size or they are in a high-risk category for future recurrence. The chance of preventing or postponing a recurrence of the cancer—and perhaps even the chance of overall, long-term survival—can be increased with the use of chemo.

The usual chemotherapy for early-stage breast cancer, while no picnic, is definitely less devastating than it used to be. Today, newer drugs reduce the nausea and fatigue. Certain drugs given during chemotherapy help the bone marrow make more new blood cells and release them into circulation. This helps prevent delays in the treatment.

Of course, chemotherapy has made wig making a real growth industry. Your bad hair day lasts about nine months. My daughter, Gail, had a lot of fun playing with my wig—or as we called it, "the muskrat." Actually, I learned to like the ease with which I could wash my "hair"—swish it in a bowl of suds, rinse it, and hang it to dry. I also enjoyed snatching it off on the hot drive home from work and chuckling at the startled expressions on the faces of other drivers.

Going through surgery and chemotherapy mobilized me, and it was easy to focus on milestones: one-third done, halfway done—finished! My eyelashes returned, and before I knew it, I was ready to donate my wig to the American Cancer Society's wig bank. Then I climbed the hill behind my house without gasping for breath, and finally I went an entire day without thinking about breast cancer.

My days now, after chemotherapy, are as precious as the glimpse of a small garden behind a city brownstone. These are good days. They have shown me, in a poignant and powerful way, that life is best lived by us all, with and without cancer, in a state of radical trust. Trust and trust and trust some more. None of us knows the limits of our days, but we do know Who limits them. And that is all we need to know.

—Suzanne Braddock, M.D.

Wind

I sit silent in the cold room, reading
when softly, a stir outside calls me away. It is the wind,
moving the frozen oaks and evergreens, pushing the
snow across the ice on the lake.
It is a sound both great and small,
the breath of God over the land
the voice of creation,
giving life to this cold, barren landscape,
to my days of terror.
I feel the power embraced in that sound,
and the joy in the force that is greater than I,
greater than cancer, greater than all the pain in all the women.

—Suzanne W. Braddock, M.D.

1

Understanding Breast Cancer

Every woman of every age needs information about breast cancer—especially in the United States, where the breast cancer rate is one of the highest in the world. If you already have breast cancer, knowledge can be your best antidote to fear and your best preparation for treatment. If you do not have breast cancer, it is your best protection.

Perhaps the most important thing to know is that every year since 1989, the death rate from this disease has declined an average of 2 percent, even though the number of cases has gradually risen. Breast cancer has also received much more publicity in recent years. More and more women are learning about this illness and their own risk. The more they know, the more they will practice self-examinations, schedule mammograms, and take care of their health. In turn, more cases of breast cancer will be detected early. That will raise the survival rate even more. Knowledge is a wonderful thing. And the best place to start learning about breast cancer is with an understanding of the healthy breast.

Breast Structure and Function

The image of the human female breast has become so glamorized and commercialized in our culture that it is easy to forget that the breast also has a job—producing milk for babies. Even a quick look at breast structure reminds us of this.

The breast is made up of fatty tissue. Breast fat contains blood vessels, lymph vessels, and fifteen to twenty rounded divisions called *lobes*. The lobes in turn are formed of dozens of smaller *lobules*, which end in tiny *bulbs*. The lobular system produces milk in response to the hormonal changes that occur after childbirth and also after a late miscarriage or abortion. The milk flows from the lobes and bulbs through narrow tubes, or *ducts*. These lead to the *nipple*, which protrudes from the center of the *areola*, the circle of darker skin at the tip of the breast.

Breast cancer isn't a death sentence. We've made so much progress in the last 20 years. In the future, I believe breast cancer will be viewed more as a chronic disease, like hypertension or diabetes.

—Kathryn, oncology RN

The lymph vessels in the breast carry *lymph*, a fluid containing white blood cells, to *lymph nodes*—small, rounded masses of lymphatic tissue. The purpose of lymph is to transport infection-fighting cells to all parts of the body, and the purpose of the nodes is to filter this fluid. Both lymph vessels and lymph nodes are located throughout the body. It is important to know about the lymph nodes near the breast, in addition to knowing about breast structure, because these nodes are usually (but not always) the first organs affected when breast cancer begins to spread.

Breast Anatomy

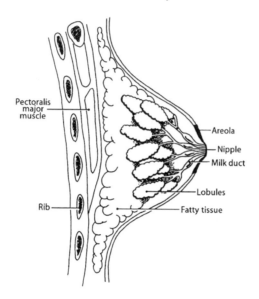

Pectoralis major muscle

Rib

Areola

Nipple

Milk duct

Lobules

Fatty tissue

What Is Cancer?

Cancer is a collection of cells growing out of control. Let's examine how this occurs. All cells in the body divide, making new cells just fast enough to replace the old ones that die. This process keeps the body's blood and organs healthy. Occasionally, however, cell division runs out of control, and the cells in a particular part of the body begin to divide too rapidly. This is called *hyperplasia.* The cells produce great numbers of abnormal new cells, which also divide at a speeded-up rate. Eventually, as more and more abnormal cells appear in body tissue, they form an abnormal growth, or *tumor.*

Some tumors are *benign*, or not cancerous. Surgically removing a benign tumor usually solves the problem for good. Other tumors are *malignant*—they are indeed cancer. Unless they are detected and treated early, they can spread from their original site to other parts of the body in a process called *metastasis*. Malignant tumors are usually treated with surgery and one or more other kinds of therapy, depending on how large they are and whether they have *metastasized*, or spread.

Types of Breast Cancer

Ductal Carcinoma

About 80 percent of breast cancers, or carcinomas, start in the milk ducts, the passages that connect the milk-producing lobes to the nipple. This type of cancer is known as *ductal carcinoma*. There are two types of ductal carcinoma: *in situ* and *invasive*.

Ductal Carcinoma In Situ (DCIS)

Ductal carcinoma in situ is a condition in which the abnormal cells have not spread through the walls of the milk ducts into surrounding breast tissue. "In situ" means "in place." In other words, the cancer is confined to the duct. This form of breast cancer is technically considered a "pre-invasive" condition—the abnormal cells have not yet become a full-blown malignancy. However, the cells can develop into *invasive* cancer and prompt treatment is important.

A ductal carcinoma in situ lesion does not feel like a lump but can occasionally be felt as a thickening of the duct. Unfortunately, only about 50 percent of DCIS cases develop the microcalcifications (clusters of tiny grains of calcium) that can

Breast with Lymph Nodes

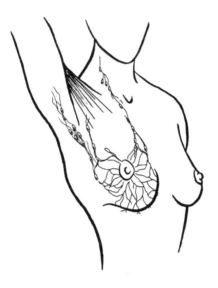

Frontal view of breast showing lymph nodes in the underarm and neck regions. The nodes filter lymph, which carries infection-fighting cells throughout the body.

be seen on a mammogram. The others either go undetected until they become malignant, or they are discovered coincidentally, when a biopsy is performed on a breast lump.

Invasive Ductal Carcinoma (IDC)

This cancer is the most common form of breast cancer. As the name suggests, *invasive ductal carcinoma* is a cancer which has invaded tissues outside the milk duct. It usually is found in a single site, rather than throughout the breast. Common symptoms include: a lump you can feel, bloody nipple discharge, or puckering of the skin. This cancer may be detected by mammogram or as a palpable lump. Invasive ductal carcinoma carries a low risk of developing in the opposite breast, at the time of diagnosis or later on. In fact, the overall risk of developing such a cancer in the other breast is only 0.8 percent per year after the initial diagnosis.

5

Lobular Carcinoma

About 10 of breast cancers are *lobular carcinomas,* cancers that begin in the milk-producing lobules. Again, there are two types: *lobular carcinoma in situ* and *invasive lobular carcinoma.*

Lobular Carcinoma In Situ (LCIS)

Lobular carcinoma in situ is a condition in which abnormal cells are found in the milk lobules, but these cells are not malignant. Rather lobular carcinoma in situ is a *marker* for cancer. Its presence means there is a higher risk that either lobular or ductal cancer will develop in one or both breasts. Lobular carcinoma in situ is rarely visible on a mammogram and is usually found during a biopsy on a breast lump. It is often found in both breasts.

Invasive Lobular Carcinoma (ILC)

When breast cancer in the milk lobules has spread into surrounding breast tissue, it's known as *invasive lobular carcinoma.* Unlike ductal carcinoma, invasive lobular carcinoma does not always produce the fibrous tumors that can be felt as a lump in the breast; rather it causes a thickening of breast tissue, making it more difficult to detect with mammography. Invasive lobular carcinoma is more likely than ductal cancer to be found in several sites throughout the breast. MRI, if available, is helpful in cases of lobular cancer to make sure all the sites are detected.

Inflammatory Breast Cancers

Other, less common types of breast cancer exist, and each carries a slightly different prognosis. Each occurs less than 1 to 1.5 percent of the time. Perhaps the most important to know about is *inflammatory* breast cancer, an aggressive form of the disease that often is misdiagnosed. Symptoms of inflammatory breast cancer usually do *not* include a lump. The cancer tends to be diffuse, beginning in the ducts and spreading rapidly through the lymph vessels beneath the skin. Signs and symptoms include:

- a sudden increase in breast size or density
- redness
- warmth
- constant pain
- *peau d'orange*, skin texture resembling that of an orange

Redness, swelling, warmth, and breast pain often lead to a mistaken diagnosis of *mastitis*, or breast infection. When antibiotics fail to alleviate the symptoms, the next step is usually a biopsy.

If you develop any of the symptoms of inflammatory breast cancer, by all means see your doctor immediately and insist on a biopsy without delay. Treatment for this condition has improved recently, but it is still an aggressive form of breast cancer.

> *For some people, getting as much information as possible helps them cope with a cancer diagnosis. Otherwise, they feel the cancer is five steps ahead of them.*
>
> —*Holly, oncology social worker*

Risk Factors for Breast Cancer

Breast cancers develop in the lobes or ducts of the breast. How and why they arise is still largely unknown, but the incidence of breast cancer is associated with many factors. Each of those listed below has been linked to the runaway cell division that in time can give rise to cancer. Some of the links are proven; others, so far, are matters of suspicion. It is important to be aware of them all.

Hereditary and Genetic Factors

In about 70 percent of breast cancer cases, there is no known history of the disease in the woman's family. In such cases, the disease is called *sporadic* breast cancer. In about 20 percent of cases, at least one relative, often an aunt or grand-mother rather than a mother or sister, has had the disease. This is called *polygenic* breast cancer. It does run in families, but most family members do not develop the illness. A family history of polygenic breast cancer increases a woman's lifetime risk from about 3.3 percent (for women with no known risk factors) to less than 8 percent—still low, overall.

In rarer cases, however—about 5 to 10 percent of all breast cancers—the disease is clearly passed on from one generation to the next in one of two genes, called BRCA1 and BRCA2, which can undergo certain *mutations* (changes) that cause breast cancer. These genes are responsible for true *hereditary* breast cancer. BRCA1 is the more common of the two. A breast cancer gene has a fifty-fifty chance of being passed on by the person carrying it. This can be the father as well as the mother, so it is possible for a woman to have hereditary breast cancer and not have a mother or sister with the disease. A woman who inherits BRCA1 (less is known about BRCA2) has a lifetime breast cancer risk of 30 to 80 percent—a large variation. Whether she develops the disease or not seems to depend on whether the cancer-causing mutation in the gene has an effect.

Environmental Toxins

In our society we are surrounded by toxins in the form of pesticides, herbicides, cleaning solvents, chemical waste, food preservatives, and even some plastics. Some of these substances, and many others besides, are known to be cancer causing, or *carcinogenic*. Others have been linked to higher rates of cancer among people exposed to them, but the link has not been scientifically proven.

Hormonal Factors

Rates of breast cancer tend to be higher among women who have been exposed to higher lifetime levels of estrogen in their bodies. This group includes women whose exposure to estrogen has been increased by:

- early onset of menstrual periods (before age twelve)
- late menopause (after age fifty-five)
- no pregnancies
- late first pregnancy (after age thirty)

The synthetic hormones in birth control pills do not appear to raise the risk of breast cancer, although cancer risks of both long-term use and early use of the pill are somewhat in doubt. In addition, it is possible that estrogen-replacement therapy, during and after menopause, might increase the risk of breast cancer. Further research on these kinds of synthetic estrogen is needed.

DES (*diethylstilbestrol*) is another synthetic estrogen. It was prescribed from the 1940s until 1971 to prevent pregnancy complications. Women who took this drug thirty or more years ago have a somewhat higher risk of breast cancer. Daughters who were exposed to DES in their mothers' wombs do not appear to share this elevated risk.

That will not prove certain until more of the daughters reach their forties, fifties, and beyond—the ages at which breast cancer is more likely to occur.

Radiation Exposure

Women who have received radiation therapy to the chest area for any reason have a greater risk of developing breast cancer. This includes women who have been treated for earlier cancers, such as Hodgkin's disease, and women who, before the risks were known, might have been given radiation many years ago for conditions such as *mastitis* (breast infection). The earlier the exposure, the greater the hazard, since studies indicate that the risk can stay elevated for thirty-five years or more after radiation exposure. If not already scheduling mammograms, women whose breasts have been exposed to radiation should begin annual mammograms ten years after the exposure. This is all the more important if the exposure occurred during puberty, because developing breasts are especially vulnerable.

> *You don't have a choice about getting breast cancer, but you do have a choice about how you deal with it. It doesn't have to ruin your life. There are things worse than breast cancer.*
>
> —Ann, 53

Nutrition Factors

There is evidence that a diet high in fat and low in fiber increases the risk of breast cancer. It has long been known, for example, that Asian women who eat a traditional low-fat, high-fiber diet have a very low incidence of breast cancer. But when these women begin eating a more Western diet—more red meat, more fat, more sugar, fewer fresh fruits and vegetables—they develop breast cancer at the same high rate as Western women.

Risks Associated with Alcohol Use

Women who drink alcohol are known to have a somewhat higher risk of breast cancer than women with no risk factors. The more alcohol consumed, and the younger the woman consuming it, the higher the risk. It is possible that an adequate intake of folic acid (400 to 600 micrograms daily) can help to counteract the risk associated with moderate alcohol consumption.

Clearly, a great many things may put women at some degree of risk for breast cancer. And even though we can't entirely control all risks, we can take steps to catch breast cancer early if it develops. The next chapter will tell you how you can do this. It will also guide you through the first things you will need to know if you are diagnosed with breast cancer.

2

Getting a Diagnosis

All suspicious changes in the breast should be investigated. The most common change is the formation of a lump. Lumps that can be felt are usually discovered by the woman herself or by her doctor during a physical examination. Most of those that cannot be felt show up in routine mammograms. Once a lump has been discovered, the next step is to diagnose it—to find out whether it is cancer. Fortunately, about 80 percent of breast lumps are not found to be malignant.

Methods of Examining the Breasts

Breast Self-Examination (BSE)

Because more than 75 percent of malignant lumps are found by women themselves, all women should perform a breast self-examination every month. This should become routine as soon as their breasts develop, or at the latest by age twenty. Because the breasts tend to swell before the menstrual period, premenopausal women should perform BSE seven days after the first day of the cycle. Postmenopausal women should examine their breasts on the same day every month, so that day becomes a reminder.

Some women avoid BSE because they are afraid of what they might find. High-risk women especially dread what they might discover. This is understandable but risky. The fact is that regular self-examination—because it is practiced so frequently— offers the very best chance of discovering a cancer while it is small and highly treatable. Finding a small tumor is much better than finding a large one.

Another reason some women are reluctant to perform BSE is that their breasts feel lumpy. This may be normal glandular tissue—ducts and lobules. Other times, women may feel benign masses called *cysts,* or *fibrocystic changes.* This condition is often (and mistakenly) referred to as "fibrocystic disease," but it is not truly a disease. Women who have benign masses in their breasts often assume they won't be able to tell when a new lump has appeared or when a lump is cause for worry. But if they examine their breasts regularly, they will learn the "terrain." They will become so familiar with the texture and the pattern of cysts in their breasts that they *will* detect changes, even small ones.

You should perform BSE in two phases, lying down and standing before a mirror. Lying down, you will examine your breasts with your hands. In front of a mirror, you will inspect them visually. Some warning signs are best discovered manually and some visually. The warning signs are:

- a lump or thickening in the breast, surrounding area, or armpit
- swelling, redness, rash, or warmth
- puckering or dimpling of the skin
- skin texture like that of an orange (called *peau d'orange*)

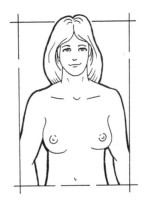

Hands at side.
Compare symmetry.
Look for changes in:
- shape
- color

Check for:
- puckering
- dimpling
- skin changes
- nipple discharge

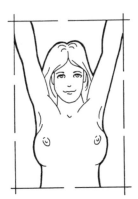

Hands over head.
Check front and side view for:
- symmetry
- puckering
- dimpling

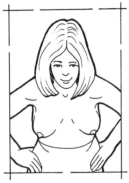

Hands on hips, press down, bend forward.
Check for:
- symmetry
- nipple direction
- general appearance

Lie down.
Place a pillow under right arm;
Raise right arm above head.
Use the pads of your three
middle fingers.

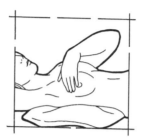

Examine area vertically from:
- underarm to lower bra line
- across breast bone
- up to collar bone
- back to armpit

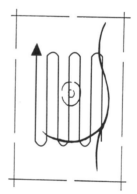

Examine entire area.
Use vertical strip pattern.
Use light, medium, and firm pressure.
Move fingers in dime-sized circles.

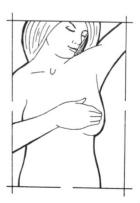

- a persistent sore or scaling of the nipple and/or areola
- drawing-in (*retraction*) of the nipple
- any change in breast size, shape, or symmetry
- pain that is persistent and focal
- persistent spontaneous bloody discharge from the nipple

To examine your breasts while lying down:

- Place a small pillow under your right shoulder, then raise your right arm and rest the back of your hand on your forehead. This position flattens the breast and makes it easier to examine.
- With the three middle fingers of your left hand held flat, use small circular motions to examine your right breast with light, medium, and then firm pressure.
- Start at the underarm. Use an up-and-down pattern, as if following narrow vertical stripes, to cover the entire breast and surrounding area—from collarbone to lower bra line to breastbone, and including the armpit.
- Repeat the first three steps, using the right hand to examine the left breast.

You can also examine your breasts with your hands in the shower or bathtub. The advantage is that soapy skin makes small changes easier to feel. The disadvantage is that the breasts are not flattened out when you are sitting or standing, so always do the exam while lying down, too. You can duplicate the advantage of soapy skin while lying down by applying a smooth lotion.

To examine your breasts in the mirror, look for any of the warning signs listed above. Do this in each of the following positions:

- with your arms down at your sides
- with both arms held straight up
- with your hands pressed against your hips to tighten the chest muscles
- bending forward with your hands on your hips

If you notice a warning sign during BSE, or at any other time, see your doctor. Do not assume that a lump can't be cancer if it moves (or doesn't move) or if it is hard (or soft), tender (or painless), or regular (or irregular) in shape. *Any* lump or thickening that was not there on your last BSE, or has not already been checked, should be examined by a doctor, regardless of its characteristics. If you are worried about a lump, insist on further imaging studies or a biopsy. You deserve a clear answer, and a doctor cannot provide one just by feeling the lump in question.

It is never safe to stop doing BSE. Women should practice it all their lives. This includes women who have had a mastectomy or lumpectomy. They should begin examining the incision right away for changes, bumps, rigid areas, or discoloration, and they should search for lumps above and below the collarbone and in the armpit. Practicing BSE on the opposite breast is extremely important, too. Survivors of some types of breast cancer are at high risk for a new breast cancer.

Clinical Examination

Women should have a clinical breast exam as part of their yearly checkup. A physician feels the breasts and breast area for thickening or lumps, checks for visible warning signs, and asks the woman general questions about breast tenderness or changes, breast care, and medical history, including family history. A trained medical person is somewhat better able to feel the difference between a benign lump and a malignant one, but a clinical exam in no way substitutes for monthly BSE. Nor, as mentioned above, can it conclusively determine whether a lump or other symptom is cancer. If the clinical exam raises suspicions of cancer, further diagnostic tests will be needed.

My diagnosis was unbelievable to me. The radiologist kept saying she was concerned about my mammogram and I kept saying it was just scar tissue from a previous biopsy. Then it dawned on me that she was trying to tell me she thought I had breast cancer.

—Kristine, 51

Mammography

A *mammogram* is an X-ray of the breast. It is performed by a technician, and the results are viewed either on film, like a photographic negative, or, using a newer technique, on a computer screen. This recent technique, called *digital mammography*, converts the X-ray images to computer code and then displays them in much finer detail than film can capture. Digital mammography also uses lower doses of radiation per mammogram. It is not yet widely available.

A *screening mammogram* is used to search for early cancers that cannot be felt, and a *diagnostic mammogram* is used to study any breast symptom, including lumps, that *can* be felt. In other words, diagnostic mammography is the first step

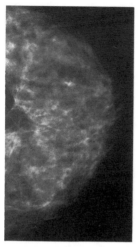

A normal mammogram.

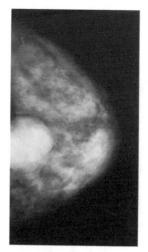

Mammogram showing
cysts with smooth edges.

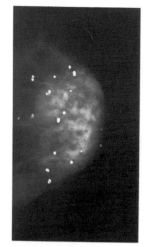

Mammogram with
benign calcifications
scattered throughout.

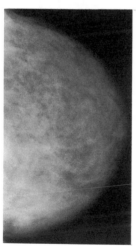

Mammogram showing a
dense pattern, usually
seen in younger women.

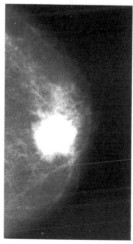

Mammogram showing
cancerous growth. Note
the irregular edges.

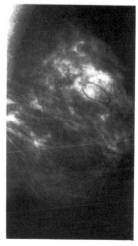

Mammogram with cluster
micro-calcifications.
These clusters are
usually benign, but may
be cancerous.

after a woman or her doctor feels a lump. Women should have screening mammograms at the following times:

- Once between ages thirty-five and forty.
- Every year after age forty. Annual mammograms were once advised only after age fifty. But the number of cases among women in their forties is about the same as among women in their fifties—and tumors often grow more quickly in younger women.
- Every year for women who have survived breast cancer of any kind.
- Every year for any woman whose mother or sisters have had breast cancer, starting ten years earlier than the age at which the youngest affected relative was diagnosed.

It is essential that an experienced radiologist reads all your mammograms and can compare your most recent films with your older ones. Mammogram results may show *microcalcifications*, tiny grains of calcium, which appear on film as small, white dots. The results may also show a star-shaped (*spiculated*) mass or nodule. The majority of masses are benign; however, mammograms can and do yield false positives—suggesting cancer when cancer is not present; or they can yield false negatives—suggesting a benign growth when cancer *is* present. The latter is a particular risk for women with dense breast tissue, because the test simply fails to "see" 10 to 20 percent of cancers in these cases. Ask your doctor or the mammogram technician if you have dense breast tissue. If the answer is yes, ask for further testing, such as ultrasounds.

Ultrasonography

Because mammography is not 100 percent accurate as a diagnostic test, other tests are sometimes used in addition. One of them, *ultrasonography*, uses high-frequency sound waves (ultrasound) to create two-dimensional images of internal body parts. These images are gathered painlessly by moving a microphone over the skin. They are then transmitted to a computer screen. Ultrasonography can detect whether a lump in the breast is filled with fluid, in which case it is a cyst, or is solid tissue, in which case it might or might not be cancer.

Positron-Emission Tomography (PET)

The *PET scan* is similar to an X-ray; however, X-ray images reveal cell structure, whereas the PET scan shows cell activity. It does this by detecting the different rates at which cells consume sugar, or *glucose*. Just prior to the scan, the patient drinks a sugar solution, and the patient's cells absorb the glucose. Cancer cells use up sugar faster than normal cells do. The more glucose used by a growth being tested, the more likely that the growth is cancer. Studies suggest that PET is highly accurate at diagnosing whether a tumor is a cancer. However, because it is a very expensive procedure, and is not available to every medical facility, it is not considered a routine test for breast cancer.

Magnetic Resonance Imaging (MRI)

The *magnetic resonance imaging* machine is a powerful magnet that acts in conjunction with radio waves to produce computer images showing differences in the number of blood vessels in various types of tissue in the body. In the case of breast cancer, the patient is injected with a dye that is picked up faster by cancerous tissue, where more blood vessels cluster, than by normal tissue or benign tumors. MRI can indeed pick up cancers in this way. However, some benign tumors with numerous blood vessels can still yield false positive MRI results. And some slow-growing cancers, with relatively few blood vessels, can yield false negatives. MRI, like PET, is expensive and not available everywhere, so it is not as commonly used as mammography or ultrasonography for detecting breast cancer. However, facilities that do have it use it regularly for this purpose.

I was so surprised that I had breast cancer because there is no history of it in my family. My first thought was, 'Oh no! My sisters are gonna kill me!'

—Joan, 47

Ductal Lavage

Ductal lavage, a newer test, is administered in only a few medical centers so far, but it is promising for women at high risk for breast cancer because it can find abnormal cells that do not show up on mammograms. It does this by examining cells from the lining of the milk ducts, which is where the majority of breast cancers begin. If abnormal cells are found, a woman might choose to take the drug tamoxifen, which has been shown to reduce the rate of breast cancer in some high-risk women by as much as 45 percent.

The procedure for ductal lavage is simple. Under mild, local anesthesia, light suction is applied to draw small amounts of fluid from the ducts to the surface of the nipple. This identifies the openings of the ducts, which are then rinsed with a saline solution introduced through an extremely fine catheter.

When the solution is drawn out again, it contains cells that are then analyzed for early signs of cancer.

The Breast Biopsy

If testing cannot rule out cancer, your doctor will order a *biopsy*—a procedure in which cells, sample tissue, or an entire lump is removed from the breast to be analyzed under a microscope. This is the only sure way to establish whether a solid lump is malignant. A woman should insist on a biopsy for any persistent or questionable lump, regardless of her family medical history or degree of risk. She should not be persuaded that a clinical examination is sufficient.

Four general biopsy procedures are used to determine whether cancer is present—two using needles and two using surgery. A surgical biopsy is called an *open biopsy*. All biopsies can be done on an outpatient basis. Needle biopsies and surgical biopsies are described below.

Before undergoing a biopsy, find out which kind you will have, how much tissue will be removed, when you will learn the results, and who will report them to you. For a tumor to be diagnosed benign, the clinical exam, the mammogram, and the biopsy all must agree on the finding. For a cancer diagnosis, a biopsy alone is sufficient.

Needle Biopsies

Fine-needle aspiration (FNA) removes cells through a narrow, hypodermic-type needle. A local anesthetic is injected, then the biopsy needle is inserted into the lump or thickening. When the plunger is pulled back, it withdraws into the syringe a small amount of fluid that contains cells from the lump. The person who examines this fluid in a laboratory must be a *cytologist*, someone trained specifically to study cells rather than blood or tissue. This procedure is the least invasive kind of biopsy, used for lumps that can easily be felt and located. If cancer is found, the result is considered reliable. If not, a larger biopsy will probably be performed.

Large-needle or *core biopsy* takes a sample of tissue from a lump. If the lump can be felt, the biopsy needle is inserted directly, after anesthesia, and withdraws a small wedge of tissue for testing. If the lump cannot be felt but shows up on a mammogram, the needle can be guided to the lump by computer images. This is called *image-guided* or *stereotactic* core biopsy. Needles are commonly guided by ultrasonography as well.

The tissue from the biopsy is studied by a *pathologist*, a doctor who diagnoses disease from tissue or blood samples. In a core biopsy, if no cancer is found, a surgical biopsy may or may not be called for. If the tumor has raised a strong suspicion of cancer during a clinical examination or imaging procedure, but the results of a core biopsy are negative, then a surgical biopsy will be performed to double-check. However, if a newly detected tumor feels benign, and also looks benign in imaging tests, then a negative core biopsy will be seen as confirming this first assumption, and no surgical biopsy will be needed.

Open Biopsies

During *incisional biopsy*, a local anesthetic is given and a tissue sample is then removed through a small incision. Results of this procedure are usually conclusive. It removes enough tissue for the pathologist to confirm or rule out cancer with confidence.

In *excisional biopsy*, the entire lump and a small amount of the healthy tissue surrounding it are removed. This procedure is used when the tumor is small and there is a possibility that all the cancer—if there is any—can be removed in this single step.

Biopsy Results

Talk to your doctor before your biopsy about when and how you will receive the results. Many women prefer to hear their test results in person, with a companion, rather than to wait for a phone call that could come at any time and under undesirable circumstances.

Waiting for test results, for information, is the hardest. When you're afraid, any wait at all seems too long.

—Ann, 53

Pathologists use the following criteria in assessing the tissue take from a biopsy:

Size of the Tumor

Small tumors measure up to 2 centimeters (less than 1 inch). Medium-sized tumors are between 2 and 5 centimeters (up to 2 inches). Large tumors are more than 5 centimeters (2 inches).

Presence of Cancer Cells in Blood Vessels or Lymph Vessels

If cancer is present in these vessels, it may be in danger of spreading beyond the original tumor.

Appearance of the Cancer Cells

Well-differentiated cells—that is, mature, highly specialized cells that do not divide or multiply very often—resemble normal breast cells and indicate a slow-growing cancer. Poorly differentiated (immature) cells indicate a more aggressive tumor.

Diploid tumor cells contain normal amounts of the human genetic material called *DNA* and have a favorable prognosis. *Aneuploid* tumor cells have abnormal amounts of DNA and are more aggressive.

I felt so afraid after my diagnosis, even ashamed, because breasts are so personal. My first reaction was to hide and not let anyone know. But it helped so much to talk to someone. Talk to other women who have been through it.

—Billie, 48

Rate of Cancer Cell Reproduction

A measurement called the *S-phase fraction* establishes, on a scale of 1 to 25, the percentage of cells that are dividing in the tumor. Results greater than 7 percent are unfavorable.

Hormone Dependency

The two female hormones estrogen and progesterone interact with cells throughout the body. The interaction is possible only with cells that have hormone *receptors*, or places where a hormone can attach to the cell. More than one kind of interaction is possible. Estrogen, for example, sometimes stimulates cell growth and sometimes blocks it. In the case of cancer, it is important to know which role estrogen plays. This can be determined by examining cancer cells to see which kind of hormone receptor, if any, is present. There are two known kinds of estrogen receptors—*alpha* and *beta*. A cell might have one, both, or neither of these affecting its rate of reproduction. Testing cancer cells for these receptors, and for progesterone receptors as well, can help doctors understand how aggressive the cancer might be and what kinds of therapy might be called for.

Staging Breast Cancer

If you should have a biopsy that shows the presence of cancer cells, you're probably going to be anxious to know the *stage* of your cancer, or whether has spread. Knowing the stage is important because it determines whether additional treatment, such as radiation or chemotherapy, is necessary. However, the final, definitive staging is determined after surgery, when the lymph nodes removed during a mastectomy undergo microscopic examination by pathologists.

Breast cancers are generally divided into five *stages*. A woman's prognosis, or chance for disease-free survival, is strongly linked with the stage at which her cancer is diagnosed.

The breast cancer range begins at stage 0, which pertains to DCIS and LCIS. As noted earlier, DCIS is more accurately called precancerous, and LCIS signifies a heightened risk of cancer. After surgery, depending on how high a woman's cancer risk already is, her doctor might suggest frequent checkups, imaging studies, and perhaps postsurgical radiation.

Stage 1

A cancer that is no larger than 2 centimeters—less than 1 inch—and has not spread to the lymph nodes in the *axilla*, or armpit.

Stage 2

A cancer characterized by any of the following: (1) it is as small as a stage 1 tumor, up to 2 centimeters, but *has* spread to the axillary (armpit) lymph nodes; (2) it is as large as 5 centimeters and *might* have spread to the lymph nodes; or (3) it is larger than 5 centimeters but has *not* spread beyond the breast or lymph nodes.

Stage 3A

Tumor or tumors either measure larger than 5 centimeters (more than 2 inches) in diameter and/or have spread to the lymph nodes that adhere to one another or surrounding tissue.

State 3B

This includes breast cancers of any size that have spread to the skin, chest wall, or internal mammary lymph nodes which are located under the breast and inside the chest.

Stage 4

A cancer that has metastasized to other parts of the body—usually the lungs, liver, bones, or brain.

Trying to stage your own cancer is strongly discouraged by health professionals. Staging is a complex process, and those who try to stage their own cancer can needlessly cause alarm for themselves and their loved ones. For example, a woman with a large DCIS, measuring 6 centimeters, may think her stage is 3A. When, in fact, the actual stage would be 0, and lifetime survival is 100 percent with appropriate treatment.

3

Coping

The moment you are diagnosed with breast cancer you're put in the position of dealing with shock and fear. And you must absorb a great deal of information you would rather not need to know. Treatment decisions must be made, followed by the phases of treatment itself. These can include surgery, radiation, chemotherapy or hormone-blocking therapy, and reconstructive surgery.

Every step of the journey brings its own demands, and each new turn affects you and the people in your life. It can all seem overwhelming. Fortunately, there are many ways to make the situation manageable. Some coping strategies are listed in this chapter, and you should be able to find some that will be helpful to you.

Learning about Breast Cancer

Take some deep breaths, gather strength, and understand that the more you learn as you go, the better you will cope. Yet the learning process itself can be stressful. You wouldn't be taking it on if you didn't have to.

When you are ready to gather information, two kinds will be helpful—information about breast cancer in general and information about your specific cancer and its location, stage, and treatment.

Meeting with Your Doctor

Your surgeon is a good first source of information about your cancer. Make an appointment to see him or her as soon as possible after you receive word of your diagnosis. Then make a list of questions to ask. Write down everything that occurs to you. If it eases your mind to research some questions on your own, before your appointment, by all means do that. The more you know before you meet with your doctor, the more you will learn while you are there. But do not expect to be on top of things yet. Take your husband, partner, or a close friend with you—someone who can take notes for you and help you remember everything that is said during this appointment. You might even take a tape recorder. If your doctor does not welcome your fact-gathering efforts, and is not willing to talk with your companion and others, find one who is more accommodating.

Questions you might want to ask your doctor are:
- What kind of breast cancer do I have?
- Will I lose my breast?
- Am I a candidate for a lumpectomy?
- What are my chances for long-term survival?
- Are further tests needed to find out whether the cancer has spread?
- When does treatment begin, and how can I know which course of treatment is best for me?
- Am I a candidate for reconstruction?

- How long will it take to recover from surgery and other treatments?
- Where can I go for more information?
- Where can I find support groups, services, or organizations that might help me deal with my feelings, my family, my fears, and my relationships with loved ones?
- Are there counselors who work with cancer patients?

Conduct Your Own Research

You will likely not get all your questions about breast cancer answered during your first meeting with your doctor. New questions will come up in the course of your treatment. Keep a list of these, and try to answer the most important question or two each day. Research as many as you can on your own. Read an article, ask other women who have been through this illness, or get in touch with your doctor. This kind of information gathering will help you feel in control and will serve your first purpose—taking care of yourself. Be cautious about comparing your breast cancer to another woman's since each case can vary a great deal.

Next to your doctor, your best sources for in-depth information about breast cancer are libraries, bookstores, and the Internet. There are dozens of books on breast cancer, ranging from the very technical and scientific to simple presentations of pertinent facts. Decide how much you want to know and then look for publications that will meet your needs.

On the Internet, you can find vast quantities of reading material. You can also find countless organizations, chat rooms, and other resources. You can even find on-line support groups and the stories of other women who have, or have had, breast cancer. These can be enormously comforting and helpful to someone just now facing it. Be discerning about information you collect and make sure it comes from a reputable source.

Meet with a Survivor

Breast cancer survivors say that one of the most important things a newly diagnosed breast cancer patient can do for herself is to meet face to face with at least one woman who has survived the disease. You might know someone personally, or your doctor might know one or two survivors you can talk to. On-line correspondence with survivors is helpful, but personal meetings usually provide more emotional support.

Setting Priorities

When you are thrown into turmoil, it's often best to meet the turmoil head-on. You can't avoid it, but you can decide what's important, what can wait, and what you can forget altogether. "First Things First" is a great motto for periods of stress and confusion. The need to prioritize forces you to think about something other than the crisis itself. Just what *is* important? What *isn't*?

Put Yourself First

Understandably, breast cancer is an emotional strain. The best thing you can do for yourself is to put your own needs first throughout the entire treatment process. Then you can help others who have suffered along with you.

This is difficult for many women. We are society's caretakers, its wives and mothers and usually its nurses, secretaries, child-care workers, and schoolteachers. Even when we occupy positions of power, we tend to put the needs of our loved ones before our own. When breast cancer strikes, we may suddenly have to reverse lifelong habits, and this can actually add further stress.

Let people close to you help. Explain to your family and friends that you must put all your energy into your treatment—not only surgery and therapies but also learning, coping, and keeping your spirits up. Tell them this will increase your chance of recovery. Explain that you need *them* to be the caretakers, but work with them to strategize about domestic and personal concerns. Chances are, those who love you will be relieved and grateful to know that there is something active and positive that they can do to help.

Minimize Outside Obligations

Life goes on, even if you aren't able to in your usual fashion. Some women continue with all their activities during breast cancer treatment; others decide to scale back a little. You may need to rethink your work and any community activities you routinely take part in. If you serve on committees or boards, or lead a scout troop, or volunteer at a local shelter, let people know that you will be out of commission for a while and find out whether someone else can fill in for you. Do the same at work—try to anticipate things that will come up and prepare for them. How many sick days

I had friends who had breast cancer and they really got me through the tough times. I would lay out all my fears and one of them would always have something funny to say about it. We would just howl. It's hard to be afraid of something when you can laugh at it.

—Ann, 53

do you have coming to you? What are your employer's policies regarding extended leaves? You might not need a long absence, but it's good to know how you could go about taking one.

Be Involved in Treatment Decisions—If You Want To

The kinds and number of medical questions that occur to you, and your approach to getting them answered, can help you find the level at which you want to be involved in your treatment planning. Bit by bit, you will discover whether you want detailed information about every procedure, medication, and treatment option—or not. You might want to learn all the pros and cons of various treatments, or you might prefer to know only what you need to know to be an informed patient. You might rather put your energy elsewhere—into meditation, relationships, gardening, or other creative or spiritual efforts. This issue could take some time to decide. Don't feel you have to rush, and don't feel that you can't change your mind. You might start out wanting to know everything and then come to feel it's no longer necessary—especially the more you establish trust and rapport with your cancer specialist.

After working with breast cancer patients for 14 years, I've found that patients connecting with other patients is the key to coping. Patients sharing their journeys is the best medicine.

—Ann, oncology social worker

Emotional and Psychological Support

In general, bear in mind that you will experience many powerful and sometimes conflicting emotions after a diagnosis of breast cancer. Acknowledge your feelings and give them room. Find people who will listen and understand, even when your feelings are difficult to describe. Do not deny your emotions, no matter how inappropriate they might seem at first. Who knows? Tuning in deeply to your wildest feelings and your most subtle ones might allow you moments of great joy, even in the midst of sorrow and anger. Life warrants all of these feelings, and more, and a crisis like breast cancer can bring all of life suddenly into sharp focus.

Not that strong emotion is inappropriate. Tears and anger are normal, so allow yourself to cry and grieve. Give yourself permission to be angry, even though other people may feel uncomfortable with anger or advise you against giving in to it. Usually, you just have to go through the anger, not around it, to resolve it. So go ahead and find the appropriate time and place to punch pillows or shout yourself hoarse. Let your anger become the energy that pushes you to learn, take charge, take care of yourself, hang onto humor and hope. Just be sure that the measures you adopt actually do *release* your anger. If you end up feeling more angry, that is another sign that you could benefit from a counselor or support group.

> *My gravy had lumps before I got breast cancer and my gravy was lumpy gravy after breast cancer. You choose your attitude. Early on, I allowed myself 15 minutes every so often to let my mind go and cry or whatever. Then I moved on.*
>
> *—Jean, 48*

No matter what outlets you choose for the feelings that will surge inside you, you will not be alone. Others will have done and felt the very same things. There are no wrong, strange, or inappropriate emotions in response to breast cancer. The only emotions you should reject are those of self-blame. You did not cause your cancer. You do not deserve your cancer.

Support Groups

Other women who are going through breast cancer can offer you validation and hope. They will understand your feelings and experience. You might find a support group vitally important, if only because it will make you realize you are not alone.

I highly recommend going to a breast cancer support group. You learn the tricks of the trade, hints for coping. No one really understands unless they've been through it.

—Mary, 43

Support groups are made up of women of all ages and from all walks of life. Most large hospitals offer support groups specifically for women with breast cancer. The women who take advantage of them report that the meetings give them strength. Hearing others express fears and share valuable information helps them realize they are not alone. Most women find great comfort in that knowledge. Unfortunately, the women who could profit most from a support group—those who are the most depressed, anxious, and fearful of the worst—often don't join one.

The National Coalition for Cancer Survivorship (NCCS) helps cancer survivors and their families start local support groups or contact existing ones. To find a local NCCS group, call the national office, listed in the Resources section of this book.

Spirituality

Some women already have a strong religious or spiritual faith when they receive the news of their breast cancer. Others begin to seek this kind of support, while some have no religious faith at all, nor any interest in exploring this very private, individual matter. If you are religious, you might find that your experience with breast cancer will deepen your faith and allow you to trust more than ever that there is a larger purpose to life. Talking with a minister, rabbi, priest, or other clergy about your illness can offer great comfort. It can also become an opportunity to learn more about what you believe, what you fear, and what your particular faith teaches about God, mortality, the self, and the right conduct of a person's life.

For a whole year, I woke up each morning and said to myself, 'You have breast cancer.' It was like being on an emotional roller coaster.

—Kristine, 51

Most of these questions concern everyone, with or without a religious faith, and so they are worth contemplating in every case. If you do not have a religious faith, you still can speak with people who do. You can also find great wisdom in the works of nonreligious thinkers, in poetry, art, literature, and nature. Find ways to look beyond the boundaries of your own life, and you will probably find comfort there. It is the kind of comfort that comes from feeling yourself small—no smaller than others, just part of an immense and very grand universe.

Meditation, Nutrition, and Exercise

One way to find a broader perspective on your individual fears and concerns is to meditate. Spending just ten to twenty minutes, twice a day, in a deeply relaxed and focused state promotes an overall sense of peace and has been shown to help the body fight the damaging effects of stress. Some women like to meditate by silently repeating the word "peace," while calmly pushing away distractions that arise in the mind. Others may wish to use a form of meditation called *visualization*, or *guided imagery*. In a calm and peaceful meditative state, they picture the body healing itself. They intently visualize their cancer shrinking, their immune cells fighting cancer cells like microscopic armies, their energy returning, their color healthy, their life back to normal.

We just want to get life back the way we knew it before cancer. Sometimes we do, but sometimes we have to change our course. Cancer turns your life, as well as your loved ones' lives, around and upside down.

—Dylece, 53

If meditation appeals to you, you can find more information about it in the usual places—books, the Internet. You might also consider looking for a meditation class or a yoga class. Some styles of yoga use stretches, movement, and body postures to promote a meditative state. Others focus on the physical aspects of yoga, and these alone can both calm and energize.

Any activity or exercise that lifts your spirits and promotes your overall health will improve both your mental and your physical well-being. Eating right is another such way to fight your cancer. A low-fat diet has been shown to decrease the risk of developing cancers. Raw foods that might inhibit cancer growth include broccoli, cabbage, brussels sprouts, cauliflower, mustard greens, turnip greens, kale, and radishes. Animal studies have shown that dietary fiber also can reduce the risk of breast cancer, perhaps by influencing the body's metabolism of estrogen, keeping it from stimulating the growth of breast malignancies.

Other studies suggest that vitamins A and C and beta-carotene protect against cancer. And more than 100 studies have shown significant decreases in cancer rates among people whose diets are high in the fruits and vegetables that contain these vitamins. Foods that contain beta-carotene include apricots, beet greens, black-eyed peas, cantaloupe, carrots, sweet potatoes, pumpkin, and spinach.

Other foods thought to inhibit cancer include fresh garlic and soy products such as soy milk, tofu, and tofu products such as tempeh. Choose low-fat tofu, however, if you're limiting your fat intake. The regular version is high in fat.

A low-fat diet goes hand in hand with exercise, which can improve both mental and physical health. Even ten minutes of exercise twice a week can increase the cells that fight off tumor cells.

Addressing the Needs of Others

Your breast cancer will affect your entire family, your friends, and even your co-workers. Your husband or life partner, especially, will experience intense emotions and fears. Your children's responses and worries will depend on their age, personality, gender, and stage of emotional development. Your friends, especially women of about your same age, will be deeply concerned about you but will probably feel a surge of anxiety about themselves as well, knowing they too could develop breast cancer.

Some people will know instinctively how to comfort you and offer help. Most will not, at least at first. Some will never be able to. Try not to judge or be hurt by people who are awkward, who avoid you, or who seem unable to deal with your illness. It doesn't mean they don't care. It's just that everyone copes differently and expresses emotions differently. There is no "right way" for the people in your life to react, even if you wish they could react differently.

Throughout your treatment, you will naturally be concerned about the feelings of people close to you. Putting yourself first does not mean you will turn off your concern for your friends and family, especially your children. Though most of your active care for the welfare of others should wait until your treatments have stopped, you will want to help in whatever ways you can from the beginning. The following sections describe what others might be going through, and how you can acknowledge their struggles.

Husbands or Partners

If your husband or partner is the strong silent type, he may hesitate to discuss his feelings for fear of burdening you. He might go into denial about your disease, or he might overcompensate by being excessively cheerful. The more you explain your feelings and needs to him, the more he may be able to face his own. You might need to give him explicit permission to open up emotionally. You might eventually have to accept that he can't do that, and can't provide the support you need, no matter how much he loves you. He might just feel too frightened, sad, angry, or helpless in the face of your disease. Letting him know that you don't blame him—and that you can seek support from friends, clergy, a counselor, or a support group—will help him cope better with his own emotions. Eventually, he might learn how to help you by helping himself. Or he might not. There is nothing wrong with a husband or partner who avoids talking about his wife's breast cancer. Everyone copes differently.

The hospital phase is a particularly difficult time for husbands and partners, who must often juggle their regular workload with new domestic responsibilities and a lot of time at the hospital. Children, friends, extended family members, and medical personnel will naturally focus on your needs. They may forget how distressed your husband or partner must be. Remind relatives and friends that they can make a world of difference by offering a kind word, baby-sitting, or otherwise sharing responsibility with your husband or partner. Looking back, many husbands and partners say they would simply like to have been asked, "How are *you* doing?"

> *When my mother was diagnosed, I was in shock. Terrified. She'd never been ill before, and I was so afraid I was going to lose her.*
>
> *—Laura, 30, daughter*

Children

Children from newborns to adults are profoundly affected by a mother's breast cancer. They all—even the smallest babies—pick up on their parents' emotions and any sense of secrecy surrounding illness. No matter what your children's ages, the best help you can give them is to allow them their natural reactions to your cancer and to talk about it to those old enough to understand. Give them just as much or little information as they can handle at their age and level of development. The following guidelines might help.

Babies and Toddlers

The youngest children often respond to parents' stress by crying more, needing more attention, eating less, and sleeping poorly. Hold and comfort them as often as possible. Try to keep them on a consistent schedule. If they have begun to talk, give them very simple information ("Mommy's sick") and prepare them for changes in the household routine ("She might have to go away for a few days to get better").

Children from Three to Six

I feel like I've been able to help others through my own breast cancer. All of my fellow teachers at our school had mammograms right after I was diagnosed. One of them found she had a malignancy in the very early stages.

—Joan, 47

At these ages, children do not yet have reasoning skills and can see things only from their point of view. They might think they caused the cancer. They might worry about getting sick themselves. They tend to fear separation, so prepare them for your absences. Because they can't understand their emotions, they might act out—throwing tantrums, hitting, pushing, crying. Try to maintain their daily routine and explain everything out of the ordinary. Comfort them, explain that they are not at fault, and acknowledge that they might feel sad or scared.

Children from Seven to Eleven

In these years, children are beginning to think logically, but they worry most about the immediate future. They will feel disrupted by your cancer and treatments. They might worry about the cost of medical care, the welfare of younger siblings, and other concrete matters. Assure them that adults will handle these. Acknowledge their feelings and fears, and always tell them the truth. If you can't promise you will recover, give them realistic reasons to hope, such as treatment advances, new discoveries through research, cases of women who have beaten the odds. At these ages, children are beginning to understand and often worry about the finality of death.

Adolescent Children

From age twelve through their teenage years, children experience rapid physical, psychological, and emotional changes that make them extremely vulnerable. Because they are trying hard to establish their independence and their own identities, and thus to separate from parents and childhood, they typically deny their vulnerability. Nothing bad can happen to *them*, only to others. A mother's illness can undermine this certainty and draw them back into childhood and dependency. Be sensitive to this. Ask them to help out, recognize that they are approaching adulthood, but remember that they still have one foot in childhood. Talk about your feelings in ways you feel teens can handle. This might prompt them to do likewise. But don't push. Sometimes just being together is more reassuring than serious talk.

Adult Children

Your grown children will want to know how to help, whether they live close by or across the country. Be aware that no matter what their age, a mother's serious illness can bring feelings of need and deep anxiety back to the fore. Some might want to take charge of your care. Welcome their concern, and share all information with them, but assure them you are capable of making all the decisions you need to. Daughters are likely to worry about their own susceptibility to breast cancer, as well they should. Urge them to perform breast self-exams and have annual checkups—but also say that your own breast cancer might make your daughters more conscientious and therefore safer.

Other Family Members, Friends, and Acquaintances

People outside your immediate family will naturally be affected by your cancer. Your parents may fear for you as if you were still a young child, and you might find your roles somewhat reversed—*you* might have to comfort *them.* Your siblings will naturally worry for you but will also feel a bit fragile themselves. If you are the first person in your generation to develop cancer, that can make them aware of their own vulnerability. If your cancer is hereditary, your sisters will have to adjust to the fact that they and their daughters are more at risk. Try to understand that their personal concerns do not diminish their love for you or their compassion for your struggle.

Both family and friends will deal with your illness in ways that reflect their personalities, character, emotional life, and just plain busy-ness. Do not be offended if some call or visit more often than others or are more forthcoming with food, favors, and willingness to talk with you. Tell them you understand how hard it is to know what to do and say. Tell them all you really need is to know that they care. You might discover that this frees them to show their concern in the ways that suit them.

Sexuality and Intimacy

Although most experts recommend resuming sexual relations as soon as possible after surgery, communication between a couple is crucial. You may fear rejection after surgery, particularly if you have had a mastectomy. Your husband or partner, meanwhile, may be reluctant to approach you for fear of causing you physical pain. Obviously, if the two of you do not share your fears openly, each can misinterpret the other's. Assure your husband or partner, when you are ready, that you are eager for the comfort and tenderness of intimacy. Tell him about any insecurities you are experiencing. Ask him whether he is feeling similar things himself.

Women often feel altered and turn away from intimacy with their husbands, but intimacy will help you get through this. My patients tell me breast cancer has made them stronger as a couple and even more intimate, on many levels.

—Holly,
oncology social worker

Keeping quiet about anxieties and letting them interfere with sexual relations will only push the fears deeper. Even before you are energetic or confident enough to resume intimacy, keep a close bond by holding, caressing, and confiding in one another. Eventually, you will be ready for sexual intimacy once more. Most husbands and partners prove to be loving, supportive, and accepting of the situation, including their mates' anxieties. If you worry that your husband or partner will find you unattractive, chances are the worry is yours, not his.

Recognizing this, your husband or partner can help put your anxieties to rest in several ways. He can remind you of triumphs in your life, times when you have been strong, resilient, or courageous. He can reminisce with you about your past together—how you met, milestones you have shared, other times when you have had to pull together to overcome problems. Sometimes focusing on another time, especially a joyous occasion such as a birth, a wedding, a promotion, or a success, can impart confidence that there are more good times ahead. And the more confident you feel, the more likely those good times become.

4

Surgery

Virtually every woman diagnosed with breast cancer undergoes some type of surgery, with or without radiation and other therapies. Overall, breast surgery is straightforward, and complications are rare. Hospital stays depend on the surgery being performed and whether reconstruction will be done immediately. Most stays are overnight; longer stays—from two to six days—are sometimes needed if reconstruction is done immediately after the cancer surgery.

Today, women with breast cancer can choose from a variety of surgical options that were not available to their mothers. Modern surgical techniques have helped many women avoid losing one or both breasts. Yet the array of options can make it more difficult to weigh the relative advantages and disadvantages. Accordingly, the greater your understanding of the options available, the more appropriate treatment decisions you'll be able to make.

Finding the Right Doctors

Like most women, you probably began your breast cancer journey with a visit to your regular doctor—either your gynecologist or your family physician. However, confirmation of cancer raises the need for a team of cancer specialists, starting with a *surgeon* who specializes in breast diseases; a *radiation oncologist*, who delivers radiation treatments; a *medical oncologist*, who delivers chemotherapy or hormone-blocking therapy; and sometimes a *plastic surgeon* for breast reconstruction.

Your regular doctor will probably help launch your search for the right medical team by referring you to a *breast surgeon*, the first specialist you need to see, both for biopsy and for later surgery. If you like this surgeon, stick with him or her; if not, ask friends, relatives, and co-workers for referrals. You can also ask your doctor for another referral, or get in touch with any number of organizations that can give you more names. These include the National Alliance of Breast Cancer Organizations (NABCO), the National Cancer Institute (NCI), and the American Cancer Society. These and other organizations are listed in the Resources section of this book with contact information.

When I walk into a breast cancer patient's hospital room and tell her I am a 10-year survivor, I can see how good that makes her feel. I remember when I was lying in my hospital bed, I didn't think anyone survived.

—Dianna, 44

Once you have found the right surgeon, he or she may in turn refer you to the other specialists you will need. The following guidelines will help you gauge whether each physician you are considering is right for you. Ask yourself whether this doctor:

- seems genuinely concerned about you, not overly clinical or detached

- is a good teacher—able to present clear, thorough explanations in language you can readily understand
- examines you thoroughly—takes a detailed history and performs a complete physical exam
- asks about your emotional state—wants to know who is helping you in your crisis and whether you have or need a support group
- gives you a realistic picture of your illness and outlook but is calm and reassuring
- has considerable experience, especially with cases like yours
- is up-to-date on the newest treatments and research
- welcomes the presence or involvement of your family members or a close friend
- supports the use of all necessary pain control
- patiently answers all your questions and does not regard any of them as unimportant
- seems alert to any confusion or anxiety on your part and draws you out as necessary
- encourages second opinions on any treatment decision

I kept a journal through my breast cancer experience to remember things so I could help others. The day of my surgery, I gave my journal to my friends and family who were with me in the hospital and they wrote their thoughts. Those have been the pages I have read the most.

—Marilyn, 61

Your spirits and confidence can be greatly influenced by trust in your medical team. So go through the questions and decide which qualities are most important to you in your physicians. Insist on these, if not in every doctor who treats you, at least in the doctor who will most often serve as the leader of your team. Medical leadership may change with the phases of your treatment—that is, the surgeon will direct the treatment, and then the oncologist will usually take over. Hopefully, your physicians will work as a team.

The team approach is especially important if your surgeon, radiation oncologist, and medical oncologist disagree on which course of treatment is best for you. This is not uncommon. Many unknowns still surround breast cancer, and these can give rise to differences of opinion. Your primary doctor should be willing to set opinion aside, support you in seeking second or third opinions, and help you go over every aspect of your care before deciding on a treatment.

Types of Breast Surgery

Partial Mastectomy

When less than the whole breast is removed during surgery, the procedure is called a *partial mastectomy*. This term refers both to *lumpectomy* (also called *wide excision*) and *quadrantectomy*, which removes a larger portion of the breast.

Lumpectomy

Considered *breast-conservation surgery*, a lumpectomy is a procedure in which only

Lumpectomy

In a lumpectomy procedure, the lump and surrounding tissue are removed.

the tumor and surrounding healthy tissue are removed. It is generally performed when a tumor is small. Breast conservation surgery is an advance- ment in the treatment of breast cancer, allowing doctors to effectively treat the cancer locally while preserving the breast. The treatment started gaining favor among women in 1990, when a National Health Institute Consensus Conference concluded that a lumpectomy, followed by radiation therapy, is as effective as a mastectomy for Stages I and II breast cancer. Subsequent studies support this concept, showing that mastectomy and lumpectomy with radiation have the same survival rates for these early cancers. Women under- going lumpectomy for invasive breast cancer, rather than DCIS, should also have one or more lymph nodes removed and check for spread of any cancer.

Quadrantectomy

A quadrantectomy removes all or a significant part of one of the breast's two upper or two lower quadrants. It is generally used when the breast is small in proportion to the tumor, or when the tumor itself is fairly large (requiring the removal of roughly one-fourth of the breast to take out the tumor and adequate margins—the edges of the tissue around the tumor). In many cases, quadrantectomy leaves the affected breast

Partial Mastectomy

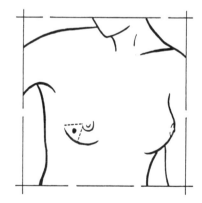

When doing a partial, or segmental, mastectomy, the surgeon removes the tumor, some surrounding breast tissue, and the lining over the chest muscles.

noticeably smaller than the healthy one. Some women later choose to equalize breast size, either by enlarging the smaller or—if they have large breasts to begin with—reducing the larger.

Total Mastectomy

Also called *simple mastectomy,* a *total mastectomy* removes the entire breast but does not remove any lymph nodes. Simple mastectomy is usually recommended for some cases of DCIS, including those where tumors are large—more than 5 cm; it is also recommended for *multi- focal* DCIS breast cancers, those in which DCIS is detected in more than one duct in the breast. It is also used as a *prophylactic* procedure, used to prevent cancer in women who have a high genetic risk or in cases where there's a high risk that a second primary cancer will develop in the opposite breast.

Total Mastectomy

In a total (simple) mastectomy procedure, the entire breast is removed, but no lymph nodes are removed.

Modified Radical Mastectomy

Modified radical mastectomy aims to remove all breast tissue (covering an area from the breastbone to the back of the armpit and the collarbone to the lower bra line) and some of the axillary lymph nodes as well.

Modified Radical Mastectomy

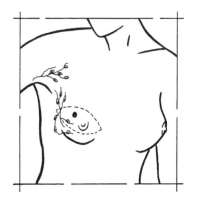

A modified radical mastectomy involves removing the entire breast, breast tissue extending toward the breastbone, collarbone, and lowest ribs; also lymph nodes in the armpit are removed and sometimes the minor pectoral muscle.

Medical reasons for modified radical mastectomy would relate to the size, stage, or location(s) of the breast cancer. Multifocal invasive cancers usually call for modified radical mastectomy. A large tumor, especially in a small breast, could likewise require a modified radical mastectomy, since breast conservation would be compromised. In some cases, however, a large tumor can be shrunk with chemotherapy or hormone-blocking therapy and then can be removed by partial mastectomy.

Both modified radical mastectomy and partial mastectomy may be offered under the same circumstances, depending on the medical facility, the nature of the tumor, and the patient's preferences. Some women choose the modified radical procedure, with or without immediate reconstruction, because they want to avoid the six weeks of radiation treatment that follow lumpectomy or quadrantectomy. Some women live in smaller communities or remote areas that simply don't allow easy access to a radiation facility. And, as mentioned earlier, some women would rather undergo mastectomy and full breast reconstruction than live with lumpectomy or quadrantectomy scars.

Other reasons for modified radical mastectomy could have more to do with the surgeon's preferences than with the patient or her particular cancer. A surgeon might prefer this procedure if he or she is completely familiar with it and prefers a tried-and-true, older approach over a newer one, even one with equally good outcomes. He or she might also simply assume that some women—postmenopausal or elderly, for example—have no real "need" for their breast anymore. Such an assumption is entirely unwarranted, since women of all ages can have many reasons for wanting to preserve their breast—reasons of self-image, womanhood, lifestyle, and general well-being. They may also prefer a smaller operation and a quicker recovery.

I had a double mastectomy and was surprised that I had very little pain. Actually, the hardest part for me was losing my hair during chemotherapy.

—Shirley, 58

Radical Mastectomy

Many years ago, a diagnosis of breast cancer automatically led to a *radical mastectomy*, a procedure that removed the entire breast, the muscles of the chest wall, and the *axillary* (underarm) lymph nodes. At the time, this extensive breast surgery was incorrectly thought to be the only guarantee of removing all the cancer.

Today however, radical mastectomy is virtually never used. Muscle is removed only in cases where it has actually been invaded by the cancer, and even then only the affected portion is taken out. Fortunately, the vast majority of breast cancer cases are discovered before that happens.

Lymph Node Sampling

The axillary (armpit) lymph nodes drain lymph from the breast and arm, so any cancer cells that are beginning to spread from a breast tumor will usually show up there first. These nodes extend in an uneven line from breast tissue below the armpit to breast tissue in the upper chest, near the collarbone. *Level I* nodes are at the lowest point in the uneven line of the axillary lymph system, *Level II* nodes are about midway along the line, and *Level III* nodes are at the highest point, above the pectoralis minor muscle. The lymph nodes are surrounded by fat pads and connective tissue.

Because breast cancer cells can travel to the lymph nodes in the under arm region, sampling these nodes for cancer is an important part of cancer staging. The presence of cancer cells in these nodes helps determine whether additional treatment is required.

Sentinel Node Biopsy

Although most surgeons still remove many lymph nodes in the armpit, a newer technique involves sampling a single axillary node called the *sentinel node*. This requires less extensive surgery than removing all or many of the nodes, and it reduces the possibility of lymphedema, a painful hand and/or arm swelling, described later in this chapter.

The sentinel node is the first node that drains the area of the tumor. The surgeon locates this node by injecting a blue dye, a radioactive tracer, or both (since they have different and sometimes complementary advantages) near the tumor. He or she then traces the substance's pathway to the lymph nodes. The first node reached by the dye and/or tracer is the sentinel node, which is then removed and examined under the microscope. If the sentinel node is free of cancer, the other nodes do not need to be removed and examined.

Axillary Node Dissection

If cancer is present in the sentinel node, a more extensive axillary lymph node surgery may be required. In this procedure, called an *axillary node dissection*, a surgeon removes Level I, Level II, and possibly Level III lymph nodes in the under arm region. The nodes are then examined for the presence of cancer cells. Today however, Level III nodes are rarely removed. The disadvantage of removing so many lymph nodes is that nerves are damaged and the risk is increased for lymphedema.

Bone Marrow Aspiration

Increasingly, bone marrow analysis is being used to help determine the stage of some cancers. At the time of the cancer surgery, doctors may withdraw a bone marrow sample from the hip, using a needle aspiration technique. Microscopic analysis of the sample is very sensitive; it can detect a single, free-floating cancer cell amid several million normal cells. The presence of such random cancer cells is called a *micrometastasis*. The cells have not yet formed a tumor, but they are likely to do so if they are left unchecked. Results of bone marrow analysis, combined with lymph node analysis and other tests, can help determine whether and what kind of chemotherapy is needed to treat a given cancer.

Surgical Incisions and Scars

Before undergoing breast surgery, be sure to consult with your surgeon about the incision or incisions that will be used.

If you plan to have a partial mastectomy, ask how the surgeon plans to minimize scarring. The shape and direction of the incision can influence whether your remaining breast tissue will pucker, whether your scar will draw the nipple out of its normal position, whether your scar will show above a bathing suit, and whether your breast will have any concave areas. If you are having your entire breast removed, and you want to have reconstruction either at the time of the surgery or later on, ask how much of your skin can be spared for the process. Also find out which direction the incision should follow to allow for the best cosmetic outcome.

Surgeons are learning more all the time about how to hide or minimize scars. Instead of studying the way an individual woman's breasts look during an examination, when she is lying down, they pay attention to how they look when she is standing, sitting, and walking. The nipple position and weight distribution are completely different in upright positions. Incision placement should reflect that in order to achieve the best surgical result.

Have someone with you before and after your surgery. My 80-year-old mother was with me and she kept saying she felt so useless because she couldn't do any housework or laundry for me. But she didn't realize what a help she was just by being there. It made a total difference.

—Marie, 45

Drains

Immediately after a total or modified radical mastectomy or axillary node sampling, the surgeon may place soft plastic tubes, or *drains*, under the skin where the incision is closed up. The purpose is to channel away fluids that builds up while the wound is healing. There might be some blood in this fluid at first, but it will soon run pale yellow, collecting in a small bulb at the end of each tube. Draining this fluid away from the wound helps prevent discomfort and infection. The drains are removed painlessly when the fluid diminishes, usually after five to seven days.

Possible Side Effects of Surgery

Pain

Most women report little discomfort after breast surgery, other than that caused by drains, incisions, or muscle manipulations (from reconstruction procedures). Your doctor will prescribe a pain medication for you to take home from the hospital, but don't be surprised if you don't need it for more than a few days. If you experience severe pain, let your doctor know. It could be a sign of *hematoma* (blood building up in tissue at the surgical site).

Anxiety and Depression

Some women experience depression after surgery, even when the outlook is positive. The body has undergone a trauma, and the biochemical reactions to trauma can produce sadness or anxiety. The mind also has been stressed, and the effects of stress can linger for some time.

Restricted Arm Mobility and Numbness

Following removal of the lymph nodes during breast surgery, your arm may be stiff for a few days to a few weeks. Physical therapy can help. You should be shown some easy stretching exercises that will immediately begin improving your mobility. Ultimately, you should have full, normal use of your arm. Even if small portions of muscle have been removed, your strength will return.

You might also experience some upper-arm numbness if, as sometimes happens, a skin nerve has been cut during lymph node removal. This can also cause tingling, sharp pains, or squeezing pressure, beginning a few days after the operation. These feelings usually subside within a few weeks. However, 2 to 3 percent of women are left with a chronic ache in the affected area.

Phantom Breast

Up to 80 percent of women who have had a mastectomy report feeling as if their breast is still present after the surgery. This perception resembles what patients feel after the amputation of a limb. If your breast tumor was painful, you might feel the "ghost" of that pain for weeks or months after your surgery. Some women report sensations that come and go for years—not painful, but reminiscent of the sensations they had while their breast was still present. These bodily sensations are all recalled by the brain, which does not forget. Such sensations do not indicate a recurrence of the cancer. Nevertheless, it is important to check with your doctor if any new or unusual pain begins, one that has not already been identified as a phantom sensation.

Lymphedema

Lymphedema is a persistent swelling in the hand and/or arm, brought on by a collection of excess lymph fluid. This condition can be caused by injury, trauma, or infection, and can develop at any time throughout your life after surgery.

Lymphedema occurs in 5 to 30 percent of women who have had lymph node surgery. The risk of lymphedema is lowest with sentinel node biopsy and highest with a complete axillary dissection.

If you develop any swelling or pain in your hand or arm, you should call your surgeon right away. If you have an infection, antibiotics, given early on, can prevent lymphedema from occurring. A specialized massage, known as *manual lymph drainage (MLD)*, given by a trained massage therapist, can help, too. Physical therapy is often prescribed as well. But the best approach is to try to prevent lymphedema. Preventive measures include care in lifting heavy objects, which can strain the arm and stimulate the production of excess fluid. It is also a good idea to avoid cuts and injuries, which can also lead to lymphedema if they become infected. Starting immediately after lymph node surgery, you should take the following precautions:

- While healing, lift nothing heavier than ten pounds with the affected arm.
- Always wear heavy gloves and long sleeves when gardening to avoid cuts and thorns.
- Be cautious using tools or objects that could break the skin—knives, nails, screwdrivers, scissors, and so on.
- Never cut cuticles; gently push them back instead. Use cuticle cream daily to prevent hangnails.
- If you plan to take a long trip by air, consider wearing a compression garment to keep the swelling down while you are in the pressurized cabin. Ask your doctor where you can obtain one.

- Ask your doctor or a physical therapist to describe post-surgery exercises that might reduce the risk of lymphedema.

For more information on lymphedema, call the National Lymphedema Network (see the Resources section).

Infection

If you notice even a slight swelling of your affected arm soon after surgery, it could be a sign of infection. If swelling, redness, or warmth occurs under the incision, notify your doctor immediately. Such infections can be serious and should be treated promptly.

Determining Prognosis

Once surgery has been performed, the breast tissue removed, including any lymph nodes, will be sent to pathologists for thorough evaluation. Based on pathology reports, physicians can determine the stage of the cancer. Accordingly, they will be in a better position to gauge your prognosis and whether you will need further treatments and how you might respond to them. Certainly, the best news you can hear is that your surgeon feels confident that he or she has found and removed all of your cancer.

In this case, you can probably expect a full recovery. Even so, you will need close follow-up, since even the best outcome cannot guarantee that every cancer cell has been removed from your body or that the cancer will not return. Getting rid of any

The word 'cancer' is the most frightening word to hear. Once you clear your mind of the fear, you can start to reason or read or do whatever gets you back on track.

—Dylece, 53

remaining cancer cells in the breast after surgery is the purpose of radiation. Destroying remaining cancer cells in the rest of the body is the purpose of chemotherapy and hormone-blocking therapy; if your lymph nodes test positive for cancer or if your tumor posed a high risk of recurrence, you may be a candidate for such treatments. Newer tests are helping to define which women with node-negative tumors are likely to benefit from adjuvant therapies and which can safely avoid them.

Because prognosis depends on so many factors—including your general state of health, individual anatomy, and responses to therapy—your doctors will not be able to guarantee what you can expect. In some cases, they can tell you what the general patterns of recovery or recurrence have been in other cases like your own.

Remember, even if you have some unfavorable indicators, breast cancer research is ongoing. New treatment techniques and findings emerge all the time, whereas current statistics are based on older ones. Continuing developments in chemo-therapy and hormone-blocking therapy are likely to yield increasingly longer life expectancies for breast cancer patients.

Questions to Ask Before Surgery

Many women feel overwhelmed by unfamiliar medical terms and decisions to make at a time when they are already emotionally overwrought. They may feel their very lives depend on the right choice, yet they also feel numb, unable to focus or make sense of things just when the need for clarity is great.

For this reason, it's a good idea to take your spouse or a close friend with you when you first meet with your surgeon.

Have your companion take notes or tape-record these conversations so that you need not grasp and remember all the new information laid out before you.

The following checklist might help you gather the information you need in order to better understand your surgery.

- What type of surgery do you recommend?
- Do you perform sentinel node biopsies?
- Will I need a blood transfusion? Can I donate my own blood for this?
- Will I need radiation therapy, chemotherapy, or hormonal therapy following my surgery?
- Can breast reconstruction be done more safely at the time of surgery, or later? Which would you recommend?
- What side effects can I expect from surgery?
- Will my surgery be done on an outpatient basis, or will I be hospitalized? If so, for how long?
- Where should my surgical incisions be made? What will my scars look like?
- Will I have drainage tubes?
- How long will I be off work?
- Will my physical activities be restricted? For how long?
- Will I need physical therapy?

Ask your doctor these and any other questions that concern you *before* you check in for surgery, but be aware that some of the answers might not be available until after your procedure is completed.

5

Reconstruction

Breast reconstruction is an option for almost any woman who has had her breast removed. In most cases, she can have the procedure either at the time of surgery to remove the breast or later—even years later. Because surgical techniques have improved steadily and dramatically over the years, more and more women today are deciding on reconstruction. In 1999, nearly 83,000 American women underwent breast reconstruction, an increase of more than 18 percent from the year before and 180 percent in just seven years.

Is Breast Reconstruction Right for You?

It has been said that mastectomy treats the disease, and reconstruction heals the mind. This is surely true for many women, yet other women feel just as healthy and strong without reconstruction. The choice is purely personal.

Some women who decide not to undergo reconstruction regard their mastectomy scar as a badge of courage. Some see reconstruction as simply conforming to the popular image of what a woman's body should look like. Women who are small-breasted sometimes feel there is little difference in their outward appearance after mastectomy. Others wish to avoid

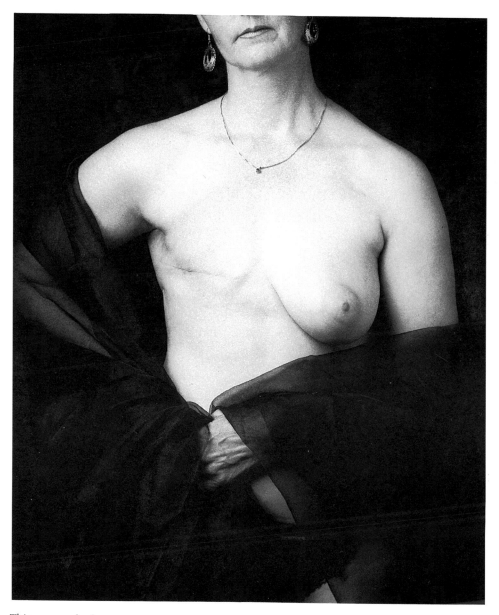

This woman had a mastectomy at age 43. She chose to not have reconstruction.

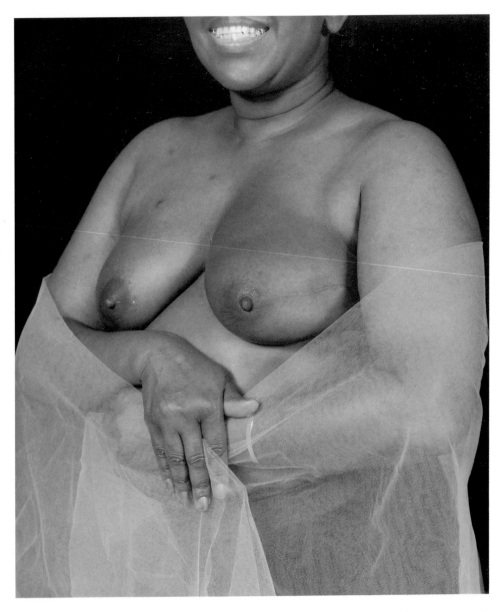

This 50-year-old woman's breast cancer was detected early. She had a lumpectomy, in which the cancerous growth and surrounding tissue were removed.

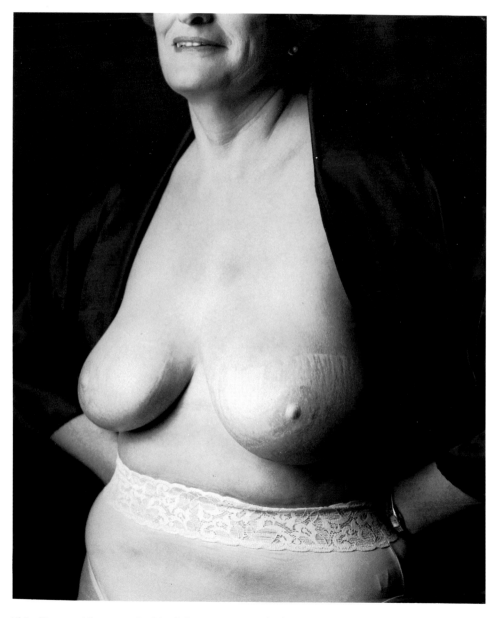

This 47-year-old woman had both breasts removed. She chose a bilateral (both sides) TRAM flap reconstruction, followed by reconstruction of the nipple and areola.

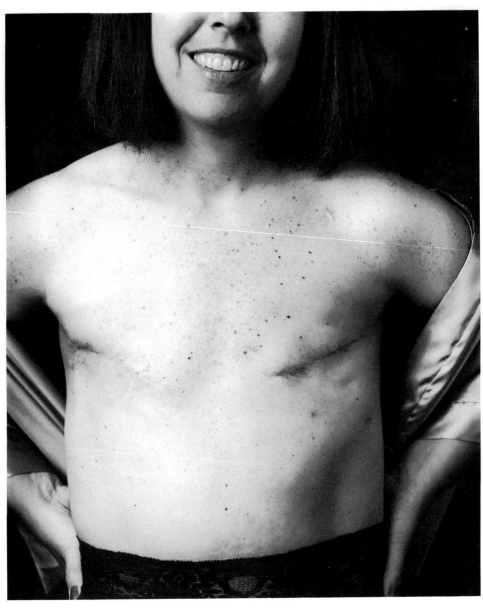

This 37-year-old woman had a bilateral mastectomy. She decided against reconstruction.

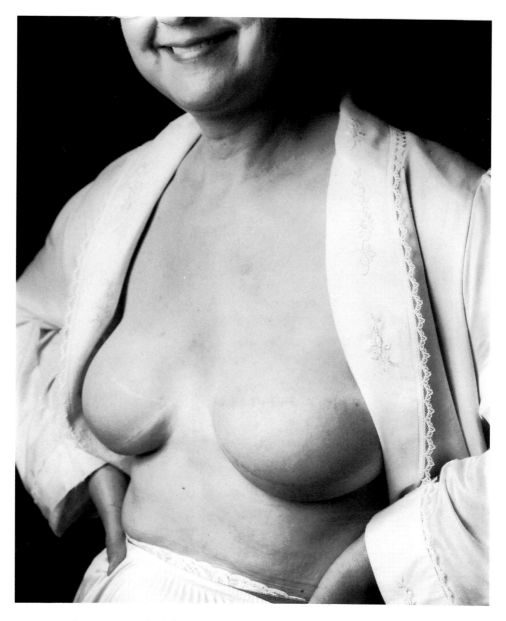

At age 50, this woman had a bilateral mastectomy. She chose to have saline implants, and is not planning to have nipple and areola reconstruction.

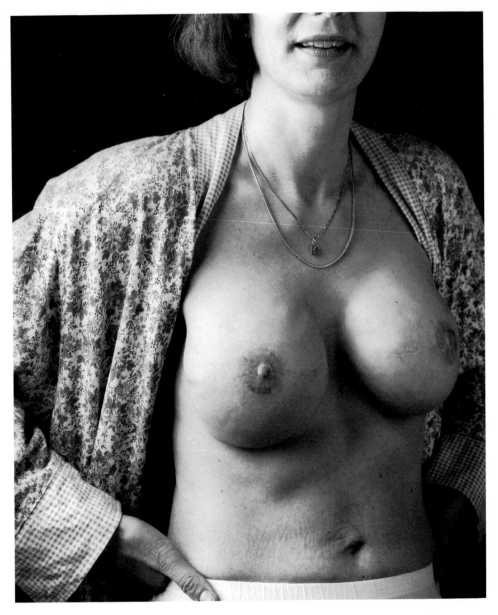

This woman, 38 at the time of her surgery, chose to have tissue expanders with saline implants. During a second procedure, she had nipple and areola reconstruction.

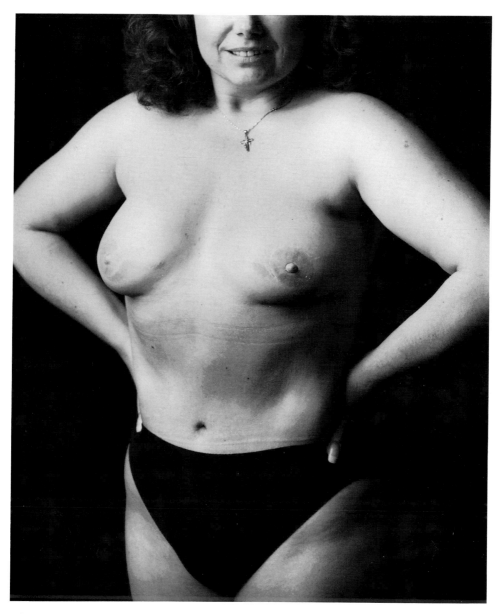

This picture shows results a bilateral mastectomy followed by immediate TRAM flap reconstruction. The nipple and areola were added later. The woman was 38 when she was diagnosed with breast cancer.

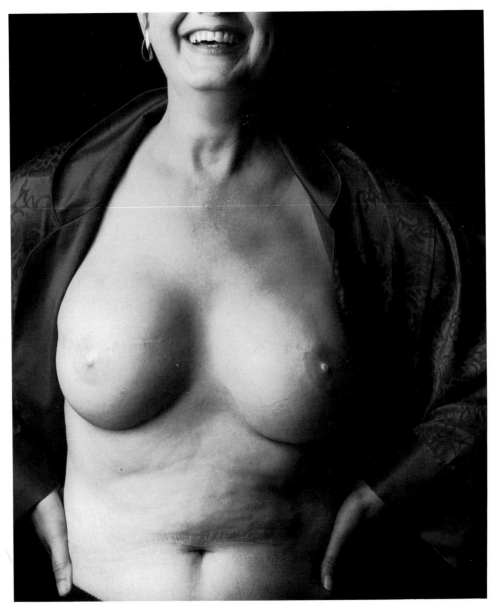

Tissue expanders were inserted immediately following this 46-year-old woman's mastectomy. Saline implants were placed six weeks later, followed by reconstruction of the nipple and areola.

any additional surgery, and are content to wear a prosthesis inside their bras. Today's prostheses are lighter and less bulky than in earlier years, and they can be worn six weeks after mastectomy when the wound has healed sufficiently.

Women who want reconstruction have at least as many good reasons as those who do not. Having both breasts may be important to their sexuality, confidence, and feelings of femininity. These women want to feel whole as well as look whole—they want to shower, dress, walk, reach, and bend with two breasts in place. If their mastectomy scar is an ever-present reminder, they may see reconstruction as the best way to put that behind them.

I was able to get through my reconstruction by telling myself, 'You can do this. You're going to look great when it's over!'

—Joan, 47

The goal of breast reconstruction is to restore symmetry or evenness to the chest wall. Because the reconstructed breast may be higher, firmer, rounder, larger, or smaller than the natural breast, the natural breast may require modification. This can be accomplished with a breast implant, a breast reduction, or possibly a breast lift.

Even though a natural appearance can be restored to the chest, the newly reconstructed breast will lack sensation. From the outside, however, the breast may feel very normal.

Making Surgery Decisions

The most important thing is to eliminate cancer from your body, and the techniques used for that can affect the methods and timing of reconstruction. For example, if you require radiation after your breast surgery, your reconstruction may be delayed until after the radiation treatments are finished. In addition, the extent of your surgery, along with the size and shape of your body and breast, will influence whether your own tissue or an implant will be used in your reconstruction.

If you are considering breast reconstruction, consult with a plastic surgeon who specializes in breast reconstruction. He or she will describe the different reconstructive procedures available and may suggest one that is best for you. You will also learn whether immediate or delayed reconstruction is better for you. Your reconstructive surgeon should consult with the surgeon who will perform your mastectomy, in order to plan a procedure that will allow the best reconstruction result. Be sure to ask your plastic surgeon to show you photographs of reconstructions he or she has performed. Try to talk with other patients who have had similar procedures.

Timely treatment is important, but I tell women they don't have to rush into treatment and reconstruction decisions within a day or two. Talk to an experienced reconstructive surgeon and to women who have had reconstruction.

—John, reconstructive surgeon

Immediate or Delayed Reconstruction?

Don't worry if you haven't made up your mind about reconstruction before your breast surgery. As mentioned earlier, in most cases, you can choose reconstruction at any time. If you do know ahead of time that you will want reconstruction, the next question is when—at the time of your breast surgery, or later? The advantages of immediate reconstruction are:

- *Financial:* Health-care costs are reduced when both the mastectomy and the reconstruction are performed in the same surgery.
- *Emotional/Psychological:* Immediate reconstruction eliminates two sources of distress—a second surgery later on, and the experience of waking from the first surgery with no breast at that site.
- *Personal:* Some candidates for lumpectomy prefer mastectomy with immediate reconstruction in order to avoid radiation therapy.
- *Geographic:* Women in rural areas where radiation is not locally available may choose mastectomy with immediate reconstruction over lumpectomy followed by radiation.
- *Practical:* Women with jobs outside the home can minimize their time away from work by consolidating the two surgeries. Women who stay at home with small children can avoid the need to arrange childcare around two surgeries.
- *Cosmetic:* As a rule, immediate reconstruction allows for a better cosmetic result because the scars are smaller.

Not every woman is a candidate for immediate reconstruction. Women in the following circumstances may need to postpone the procedure:

- Those who will need radiation therapy following breast surgery.
- Those with advanced breast cancer.

- Those whose emotional, psychological, or physical health is compromised. This includes women with serious health concerns in addition to their cancer, or women facing serious difficulties such as divorce, bereavement, unemployment, or financial crisis.

The biggest advantage of delayed reconstruction is time. For many women, the decision-making process for breast surgery alone can be exhausting. Putting reconstruction off for a while allows them to consider their options carefully, to recover from the mastectomy, and even to see how they feel without reconstruction. If you decide to delay either the decision or the procedure, remember to consult with your surgeon about the strategic placement of the mastectomy incision.

All reconstruction options are available even with chemotherapy and radiation. Reconstruction is a personal decision and therapies don't affect that decision.

—Stephen, medical oncologist

Reconstruction Options

Thanks to refinements in breast reconstruction techniques over the last decade, women can now choose from a variety of reconstructive options. Procedures that use a woman's own skin, fat, and muscle have become more and more common, and the resulting new breast usually feels and looks more like a natural breast than one formed with an implant. For example, "skin-sparing" surgery, usually done with immediate reconstruction after mastectomy, involves making incisions that minimize scarring and leaving a "pocket" of skin to be used in shaping a new breast. Reconstructive tissue can be taken from the buttocks, outer thighs, or back, and most commonly the lower abdomen. The reconstructed breast will still have little sensation, but because it is made from your own body tissue, it is more likely to match your opposite natural breast.

Reconstruction with Implant

Reconstruction with implants has two major advantages: It requires less surgery and a shorter recovery time than procedures using your own body tissue. A breast reconstructed with an implant usually feels firmer than the opposite breast, and the reconstructed breast will tend to stay firm and keep the same shape even though the other breast will change with age.

Even if you're not having reconstruction, you may want to have a plastic surgeon do the surgery or work together with your surgeon. The plastic surgeon will help you look nicer after the surgery.

—Anna, 45

There are potential, occasional risks associated with implants. The implant can develop a layer of scar tissue around it, making it feel somewhat rigid. Infection rates are very low, but if infection does occur, the implant needs to be removed. Occasionally, implants develop some wrinkling, which may be visible. The implants may leak and require replacement, but leakage should not create a health hazard. Implants should last at least ten years.

Implants available today are filled either with saline (a salt-water solution similar to the body's own fluids) or with silicone gel. There was considerable controversy in the early 1990s over the use of silicone for breast implants. As a result, regulations have been in place since 1992. Silicone has not been banned, because studies have not shown that it is harmful. But today, silicone implants are available only to women with breast cancer, breast injuries, or breast deformities.

The debate continues. However, most physicians do not see health problems in their patients with silicone implants. Doctors report that complaints, when there are any, are nearly always about the appearance or firmness of the implanted breast or about leakage—but not about illnesses caused by the silicone.

Implant with Tissue Expansion

If you decide on breast reconstruction using an implant, your first step might be tissue expansion, a method of gradually stretching the skin and chest muscle under which the permanent implant will be placed. This process can get under way at the time of your mastectomy or later. A temporary, expandable implant will be inserted under the skin and chest muscle during a procedure that usually takes from forty-five to ninety minutes. Sterile saline is added to the expander each week through a valve under the skin (there are no external tubes). The injections are normally painless because the skin is

Implant

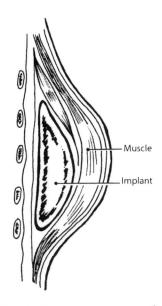

An implant is the most common method of breast reconstruction. A tissue expander, filled gradually with saline, is used to stretch the skin so it will accommodate the insertion of an implant.

usually numb for a period of time after surgery. The gradual stretching of skin and muscle in most cases involves only mild discomfort for a day or so after fluid is added. When the expander has reached the desired size, and the surgeon has enough skin to work with, he or she will replace the device with a permanent implant in a second, outpatient surgical procedure. The entire process usually takes about three months. You may not need tissue expansion if your opposite breast is small and enough skin remains on the reconstructive side to accommodate an implant of about the same size.

Tram Flap

The TRAM Flap

A TRAM flap (*Transverse Rectus Abdominis Myocutaneous Flap*) is one that uses a "flap" of abdominal skin, muscle, and fat to create a new breast. The base of the flap remains connected to the abdomen, keeping the blood supply intact and ensuring that all the tissues stay alive.

During the procedure, the flap is transferred to the breast area through a "tunnel" created under the skin by the surgeon. To accomplish this, the surgeon disconnects the lower end of the transverse rectus abdominus

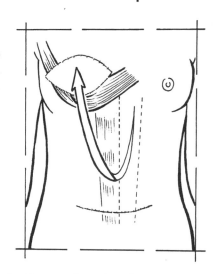

In this procedure, skin, fat, and muscle from the lower abdomen is used. The rectus muscle is disconnected, but left anchored to the rib cage. Then, the skin and fat, which remains attached to the muscle, is rotated upward to form the breast. The fat tissue in the flap helps form the new new breast.

71

(a long narrow muscle that extends from the rib cage down to the lower abdomen) from the pelvic bone, leaving it attached at the lower ribcage. This allows the flap to be turned around and pulled through the tunnel to the breast area.

Then, once the flap is drawn up to the chest, it is shaped much like the opposite breast. One of the advantages of this procedure is that, because the underlying abdominal fat is similar in consistency to the fatty tissue of a normal breast, the new breast can look and feel very natural.

The disadvantage of the TRAM flap procedure is that it leaves a long scar below the navel, and is a more extensive operation than an implant procedure. The operation usually takes three to five hours, and recovery time is normally six to eight weeks. Blood transfusions are rarely necessary during this operation, but just in case, talk to your doctor about donating your own blood in advance. In addition to having a newly reconstructed breast, the patient receives a cosmetic bonus—a flatter stomach; the tissues removed for the flap are the same ones removed for a so-called "tummy tuck."

Major complications with TRAM flaps are infrequent if the surgeon is experienced with the operation, the patient is well selected, and the operation is well executed. Potential complications include, but are not limited to, infection, complete or partial loss of the transferred tissue, and abdominal wall weakness.

TRAM flap reconstruction will probably not be an option for you if any of the following apply:

- you are obese or very thin
- you have abdominal scars from a previous surgery
- you are a heavy smoker

- you have diabetes or other blood vessel disease
- you have pre-existing lung or heart disease

Latissimus Dorsi Flap

In this procedure, part of the large flat muscle (along with the skin covering it) on the back, under the shoulder blade—the *latissimus dorsi*—is moved to the chest to form a new breast. If the muscle does not provide sufficient tissue, an implant might also be used. This method of reconstruction may be used when tissue transfer from the abdomen is not possible—for instance,

Latissimus Dorsi Flap

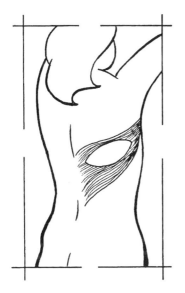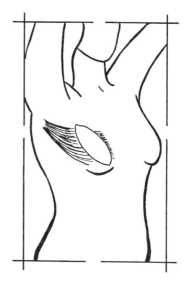

In this procedure, the latissimus dorsi muscle in the back is disconnected, but stays attached at the armpit. The skin and fat, attached to the muscle, is pulled around to form the breast. This procedure usually also requires an implant.

73

if there is scarring from earlier abdominal surgery or if the abdomen has too little fat. It is also used when more skin is necessary to cover an implant and the patient doesn't want to use the tissue-expansion technique.

The advantage to this procedure is it leaves a smaller breast scar; however one disadvantage is that it leaves a long scar on the back.

Gluteal Flap

In this surgery, the tissue used for reconstruction is taken as a wedge from one of the buttocks. The procedure is longer and more complicated than for a latissimus dorsi flap, because the blood vessels must be cut and then reattached microscopically. For this reason, the gluteal flap may be used when *neither* a TRAM flap nor a latissimus dorsi flap is possible. Its advantages are the same as for a TRAM flap—a natural-looking, natural-feeling breast that will gain and lose weight with the rest of the body. Its major disadvantage, apart from the surgical complexity, is that it leaves a significant scar where the flap of tissue has been removed. It is not widely used.

Nipple and Areola Reconstruction

If you decide you want nipple and areola reconstruction, you will probably need to wait at least six to eight weeks after breast reconstruction. Your surgeon will not save the nipple and areola from your removed breast, because this tissue could contain cancer cells. Instead, the surgeon will usually create a new nipple from the skin and fat of the central portion of the reconstructed breast. The areola can be reconstructed with a skin graft from the abdomen, inner thigh, or labia. Both the nipple and areola can be tattooed for a good color match, if necessary. Both can be reconstructed on an outpatient basis.

Insurance Coverage

Insurance companies are required by law to pay for reconstruction of the surgically treated breast and any surgery necessary on the opposite breast in order to obtain the best possible result. This is a result of The Women's Health and Cancer Rights Act passed in October 1998.

Many insurance policies will also pay for physical therapy after surgery. This is occasionally necessary to restore full arm movement after mastectomy, with or without reconstruction. Usually, simple stretching exercises prescribed by your surgeon are sufficient to relieve stiffness. This is a great improvement over the days when mastectomy routinely removed the muscles of the chest wall. Rehabilitation then was complicated, time consuming, and not entirely successful.

Breast Forms or Prostheses

If you have decided against reconstruction, at least for the present time, you have two options—to wear or not to wear a prosthesis. Some women feel comfortable making no effort at all to disguise the fact that they have had a mastectomy. They may be small-breasted to begin with, or they may wear loose clothing. They may just want to avoid the trouble of finding and fitting a prosthesis and wearing it every day. Or they might feel that they want to make a statement—they want others to see the reality of breast cancer and its effects.

Nevertheless, most women who decide against reconstruction prefer to look more natural when they are dressed, and there are many attractive alternatives available to them. Your surgeon or hospital can put you in touch with someone to help you choose a prosthesis, starting with one to wear home immediately after your surgery. This volunteer might represent a manufacturer of breast forms, or she might come from the American Cancer Society's Reach to Recovery program, which trains breast cancer survivors in supporting other women with the disease. She can visit either before or after your surgery to present and demonstrate various prostheses, discuss their pros and cons, and tell you what they cost and where you can purchase them.

I chose a TRAM flap because I didn't want an implant. It's a decision you should make on your own. If I had it to do over again, I would make the same decision, even though it's a longer recovery.

—Julianne, 54

Today's breast forms are not only more convenient and comfortable than older ones but can more easily be matched to your other breast in size, weight, and appearance. Some attach to the chest wall with the help of a small piece of Velcro-like fabric that can remain painlessly in place for several days or weeks. Others attach inside a bra. There are special prostheses for swimming or sports, and some companies sell swimsuits and other revealing garments designed for women who have had mastectomies. Prostheses are sometimes covered by insurance, so you should be sure to check. They are available in specialized lingerie shops, where you can be fitted for one that is precisely the right size and shape for you. You can also obtain them through mail-order catalogues or on the Internet.

6

Chemotherapy and Hormone-Blocking Therapy

Chemotherapy and hormone-blocking therapy are *systemic* treatments, which means the treatments are given in the form of drugs that travel throughout the body. They are also called *adjuvant* (auxiliary) therapies because they support and enhance the effects of surgery and/or radiation. Chemotherapy drugs are *cytotoxic*, or poisonous to cells. Their purpose is to destroy undetectable cancer cells—also called *micrometastases*—that might have spread to areas beyond the location of the original tumor. Drugs used in hormone-blocking therapy keep certain cancer cells from reproducing by depriving them of the hormones they depend upon. In cases where cancer cannot be removed surgically, these drugs may be used with the intent of shrinking a tumor.

Studies show that long-term survival rates increase significantly when local cancer therapies (surgery with or without radiation) are quickly followed by systemic ones (chemotherapy, hormone-blocking therapy, or both). However, if a cancer is caught very early, adjuvant therapies may not be required at all.

Finding the Right Specialist

It is important that adjuvant therapies (especially chemo-therapy) be administered by an expert—a physician called a *medical oncologist,* who specializes in systemic cancer treat-ments. Your surgeon will probably refer you to a medical oncologist if one is available in your area. This physician should have the following qualifications:

- He or she should be board certified in this specialty, meaning that he or she has taken the necessary training and has passed rigorous examinations in medical oncology.
- Or, he or she should be a board-certified *hematologist,* a specialist in the treatment of blood disorders.
- And, he or she should have considerable experience in the treatment of breast cancer with adjuvant therapies.

This specialist should be someone who inspires your confi-dence, listens carefully to your questions and concerns, and puts you at ease.

To ensure the best possible treatment, come to each appointment with a list of your questions. Take a list of all your medications as well, including birth control pills, vitamins, and herbs. Even over-the-counter drugs, such as aspirin, ibuprofen, sleep aids, or cold medicines, are important for your doctor to know about.

When Are Adjuvant Therapies Used?

Chemotherapy

The decision about when and whether to use chemotherapy is based on such factors as the type and aggressiveness of the tumor and the age and underlying health of the patient. In general, chemotherapy is usually recommended when cancer has spread from the breast to the underarm lymph nodes, or when a tumor is larger than 1 centimeter, whether the nodes are cancerous or not. When tumors are smaller than 1 centimeter, and the nodes show no evidence of cancer, chemotherapy should be considered on a case-by-case basis.

Chemotherapy drugs are highly toxic. They act against all cells that divide rapidly—not only cancer cells but normal cells that reproduce at a rapid rate. Normal cells that divide rapidly include hair cells, gastrointestinal cells, and bone marrow cells. Although the prospect of hair loss is very upsetting to most women, hair grows back without lasting damage. Gastrointestinal cells likewise regenerate. However, bone marrow must be carefully monitored and given time to regenerate *between* chemotherapy treatments.

Hormone-Blocking Therapy

When the growth of a tumor is stimulated by the female hormones estrogen or progesterone, hormone-blocking drugs can deprive the cancer of these needed nutrients. The drugs attach to the cancer at sites called *hormone receptors*. Hormone-blocking therapy is generally given whenever hormone receptors are present, regardless of tumor size or lymph node involvement.

Premenopausal and Postmenopausal Patients

In general, it is more common for premenopausal women to receive chemotherapy rather than hormone-blocking therapy, because their tumors can be especially aggressive and such tumors tend to lack hormone receptors—that is, they are not dependent on hormones to grow. Younger women also have a longer life expectancy than older women, and this means more years in which cancer could recur. Chemotherapy can help reduce this long-term risk.

When I was diagnosed, tears came to my eyes, but I was more worried about my husband and two boys. How would they handle it if something happened to me? My main thought was helping them get through this.

—Julianne, 54

Postmenopausal women are more likely to receive hormone-blocking therapy for the opposite reasons— because their tumors are often slow growing and do depend on hormones.

However, the two kinds of therapy are given together when all the conditions that call for both are present. For example, a woman with a hormone-dependent cancer that has spread to the lymph nodes or is larger than 1 centimeter is likely to receive chemotherapy followed by hormone-blocking therapy, whether she is premenopausal or post-menopausal.

Neoadjuvant Therapies

Although adjuvant therapies usually follow surgery, they are sometimes administered beforehand to shrink a tumor to operable size. They are then referred to as *neoadjuvant* therapies.

Hormone-Blocking Drugs

As mentioned earlier, this class of drugs deprive tumors of the estrogen they need by blocking either the hormone receptors or the body's production of estrogen. These drugs are capable of acting against cancer cells without harming cells in the rest of the body. For this reason, hormone-blocking therapy is the easiest adjuvant therapy to tolerate.

So far, less is known about progesterone receptors and methods of blocking that hormone. However, women whose tumors have receptors for progesterone, but not estrogen, still appear to benefit from the estrogen-blocking therapies.

Hormone-blocking therapy increases survival rates by reducing the possibility of the same cancer recurring or a new cancer developing. Its benefits have been shown to continue at least fifteen years after the five-year treatment period, with close follow-up care. This applies in all cases, but of course if the cancer is caught at an early stage, long-term survival rates are higher to begin with.

Tamoxifen

The drug most commonly used for hormone-blocking therapy is tamoxifen (trade name Nolvadex), which belongs to a category of drugs called *SERMs* (*selective estrogen receptor modulators*). It works by blocking the hormone receptors on cancer cells and depriving the cells of the estrogen they need to grow. There is evidence that tamoxifen does this by becoming incorporated into the cell and directly preventing the next cycle of cell division. The result is not just a temporary block but actual cell death.

In order to maximize the chance that as many remaining cancer cells as possible will be destroyed by tamoxifen, the drug is usually given in a daily dose of 20 milligrams for five years. It is taken by mouth. Tamoxifen therapy usually begins within four weeks after surgery or chemotherapy, or immediately after radiation therapy has ended.

Even though tamoxifen acts against estrogen in cancer cells, it acts very much *like* estrogen in heart and bone tissue. So, although it may cause some menopausal symptoms (such as vaginal dryness, fatigue, depression, hot flashes, weight gain, and insomnia), it also may protect against osteoporosis and coronary artery disease. Memory loss also is associated with tamoxifen use. However, this may not be caused directly by the drug but by menopause, which is known to be accompanied by memory loss.

> *Ask a lot of questions and take a big part in your treatment. Get to know the nurses and joke around with your doctors. I can't emphasize enough the importance of laughter!*
>
> —*Sandy, 44*

A very low risk of uterine cancer has been linked to tamoxifen, but usually when the drug is used for more than the five-year treatment period that is now standard. Tamoxifen also may have an effect on the eyes, including the possible formation of cataracts, so regular eye examinations are recommended. Ask your doctor for a comprehensive list of possible side effects. Most are mild and easily managed.

Other SERMs

Tamoxifen, the first SERM to be developed, has been studied and used against breast cancer for the past twenty years.

Other SERMs are now in use or undergoing research as scientists attempt to develop new ones that offer the benefits of tamoxifen but without the side effects. One of these, raloxifene (Evista), has been approved for the prevention of osteoporosis and is currently undergoing study for breast cancer.

Several other SERMs are being studied or have recently come into general use. Goserelin (Zoladex) suppresses estrogen production in premenopausal women. It causes temporary menopause, with menopausal symptoms being the only side effects. The drugs anastrozole (Arimidex), letrozole (Femara), and exemestane (Aromasin) block estrogen production in postmenopausal women by inhibiting the enzyme *aromatase.* Aromatase converts other hormones to estrogen and is the principal source of estrogen after menopause. Arimidex is used either as a first hormone-blocking treatment or when other drugs, such as tamoxifen, have not fully halted the disease. Its side effects can include fatigue, hot flashes, nausea, back pain, bone pain, some hair loss, and blood clots. Similarly, Femara and Aromasin have proven effective against tumors that resist tamoxifen. Not everyone taking these drugs will experience side effects; however, a possible side effect of Femara is shortness of breath. Possible side effects of Aromasin include: cough or hoarseness, shortness of breath, fever or chills, increased blood pressure, lower back or side pain, and swelling of hands, lower legs, or feet.

Chemotherapy is the finishing touch that provides a little extra reassurance against cancer cells.

—Lynn, 33

Chemotherapy Drugs

Chemotherapy today is a far less frightening prospect than it was in the past, thanks to a wider selection of drugs, a deeper understanding of how they act against cancer, and a more precise calculation of timing and dosages. There are still significant side effects from chemotherapy, but many of these can be moderated by medication.

Different categories of chemotherapy drugs behave differently against cancer cells, and so they are usually used in combination to maximize their overall effects. The most commonly used kinds of drugs work as follows:

- *Alkylators* inhibit cell division and growth by replacing hydrogen in certain cell molecules. The drug cyclophosphamide, sold as Cytoxan (C), is the most commonly used alkylator.

- *Antimetabolites* cause a cell to die at the moment when it is ready to divide. Methotrexate (M) and 5-fluorouracil (F) are standard drugs in this category.

- *Antibiotics* prevent the genetic material in a cell from reproducing. Doxorubicin, sold as Adriamycin (A), has been used for this purpose for many years, but epirubicin (E) has milder side effects and is now being used more often.

- *Antimicrotubules* directly kill cancer cells with relatively little damage to normal cells. These drugs are called *taxanes* (T). The ones used most often are paclitaxel (Taxol) and docetaxel (Taxotere).

Although other chemotherapy drugs are available, and many combinations are possible, standard treatment usually involves either CMF (Cytoxan, methotrexate, 5-fluorouracil) or AC (Adriamycin, Cytoxan) followed by T (one of the taxanes).

Every chemotherapy drug has specific, individual side effects, and these can be counteracted or moderated in a variety of ways. Be sure to ask your doctor about measures you can take. He or she might advise, for instance, drinking lots of water, avoiding certain foods, or taking medications that can reduce the side effects.

Administration and Dosages

Chemotherapy drugs are sometimes taken by mouth. In most cases, however, they are injected or *infused* (slowly "dripped") directly into a vein through an intravenous, or I.V. tube. Less commonly, a small *port*, or entry, is surgically implanted just under the skin. From the outside, it looks like a tiny button. The port is attached to a tube leading directly to a large vein, and it remains in place until all chemotherapy treatments are finished. The port is often more convenient for patients and eliminates the need for inserting IVs during every round of chemotherapy. This method may be used when conditions such as obesity or swelling make it hard to find a vein. Chemotherapy must always be given by an experienced, thoroughly trained oncology nurse, so each treatment requires a visit to the oncologist's office.

I used to whip off my wig on the hot drives home from work and enjoy the astonishment on the faces of other drivers.

—Suzanne, 58

Dosages of chemotherapy drugs are determined individually for each patient. In general, medical oncologists want each treatment to kill as many cancer cells as possible without putting the patient at risk. The range of acceptable dosages is small, but within that range there is room for differences of opinion. Some oncologists prefer to give the highest acceptable dosages less often; others prefer to give lower dosages more often. This is one reason treatments might be given weekly, every other week, or even monthly. Other reasons have to do with the nature of each drug and drug combination.

Timing of Chemotherapy Cycles

The earlier chemotherapy is given, the fewer cancer cells it will have to attack and the better its success will be. Usually, it begins three to four weeks after surgery. It is given in weekly to monthly cycles over the course of three months to as long as a year. In most cases, treatments are finished in three to six months.

So often, women think they have to do everything. My advice: if people offer help, be gracious and accept it. It's important to be good to yourself, especially during chemotherapy.

—Kathryn, oncology RN

There is good reason for chemotherapy drugs to be given in cycles. First, there is no way to detect cancer cells that might remain after surgery or radiation, because it is not possible to examine every part of the body for micrometastases. Second, it is not possible for a single, high dose of chemotherapy drugs to kill every cell at once—that would be far more toxic than a patient could withstand. It would also not be feasible, since the drugs generally kill cells only while they are dividing.

Thus the best way to administer chemotherapy is in "waves." The first wave of treatment will kill many cells that are just then in the process of dividing. It will miss cells that are at rest but will kill some of these in the next wave. The cycles of treatment continue with the intent of wiping out as many remaining cancer cells as possible. The number and duration of "attacks" depend on the drugs being used, their dosages, and the stage of the cancer.

Side Effects of Chemotherapy

Despite the many advances in chemotherapy over the years, you will probably feel nervous about its side effects. It might help if you remind yourself that these are only temporary. Side effects also vary widely from person to person and drug to drug. Just because an acquaintance had problems with nausea and hair loss doesn't mean you will. You might be on a different chemotherapy regimen and schedule; you might react differently to the drugs being used; and you might be given different medications to control your side effects.

> *Losing my eyebrows was harder than losing my hair. I don't know if other people noticed it, but I did. My hair grew back curly and I love it. I'm going to keep it short and curly.*
>
> —*Ann, 53*

Lowered Blood Count

Bone marrow produces red blood cells, white blood cells, and platelets. When chemotherapy damages bone marrow cells, production of all three blood components is slowed. This affects the body in a different way for each component.

Red blood cells carry the oxygen that gives the body fuel for energy, so a reduction in red blood cells causes fatigue. You might notice some shortness of breath as well.

White blood cells fight infection, and when they are diminished the risk of infection increases. If your white blood cell count gets dangerously low, your doctor might briefly postpone your chemotherapy treatment or lower your dosage. Or, he or she might recommend an injection of a growth factor (Neupogen) that causes bone marrow to produce and release more white blood cells. This should enable you to keep to your normal chemotherapy schedule. If you notice signs of infection, such as fever, redness, pain, or swelling, report them promptly to your medical oncologist.

When blood platelets—cells that aid clotting—become low, you may bruise easily. If this happens, or if unusual bleeding occurs, notify your doctor. To guard against dangerously low blood counts, your blood will probably be drawn and tested every time you go for a treatment.

Nausea

Nausea has not been completely eliminated as a side effect of chemotherapy, but most of it can be controlled by prescription drugs. Some drugs are taken orally, others are injected. The drugs used most often for nausea are Zofran, Compazine, and Phenergan. Patients who do experience nausea say it usually lasts a few days and then subsides.

Eating slowly, and eating small amounts of food at a time—especially dry foods such as toast or crackers—may help. In particular, health professionals recommend not eating heavily right before a treatment.

Hair Loss

Many women dread losing their hair more than any other side effect of chemotherapy. They are usually reassured to know that this effect is not permanent. Not only will their hair grow back completely, it may even be thicker, curlier, or a slightly different color than it was before. Some women don't experience complete hair loss at all—they notice only a thinning of their hair. Either way, this side effect usually starts two or three weeks after chemotherapy begins.

Before your treatment begins, you might want to buy or reserve an attractive hair-piece that matches your hair color and is cut and styled to your liking. Being prepared for hair loss can help you manage this side effect better if it does occur. If you think you will feel uncomfortable wearing a wig, try stocking up on hats, scarves, and turbans. Many women get very inventive with head coverings and take pleasure in drawing compliments.

If you do lose your hair—including your eyebrows, eyelashes, and body hair—it will grow back within three to five months after chemotherapy. Regrowth sometimes begins even before chemotherapy has ended. A program called "Look Good...Feel Better" puts women in touch with cosmetologists who provide free advice on makeup and wigs. For more information, see the Resources section at the back of this book or call the nearest American Cancer Society office.

> *I had two rounds of chemotherapy and radiation. But every day puts you in a better place. The greatest lesson I learned was that hard times don't last. You will feel better. Things will get better.*
>
> *—Ann, 53*

Memory Loss

Some women who have undergone chemotherapy report a condition often referred ro as "chemo brain." These women report such symptoms as memory loss, problems with attention or concentration, and brief episodes of confusion. These symptoms, which can be long-term, are most often associated with the chemotherapy agents in the taxane class. Research into this problem is ongoing.

Fatigue

Women typically experience fatigue during the course of their chemotherapy treatments. A flexible schedule helps. If you find yourself tired late in the day, try making time for a nap before dinner.

Fatigue may increase as the months of chemotherapy progress, and it may persist for a few months up to a year after treatment ends. In cases where fatigue is caused by low blood counts, drugs that stimulate production of red or white blood cells can help. Two such drugs are epoetin alfa (Procrit), which is a synthetic form of the human protein erythropoietin, and filgrastim (Neupogen).

Menopause

Some women stop menstruating during chemotherapy and also may experience the night sweats and hot flashes common in menopause. Other menopausal symptoms include vaginal dryness, fatigue, depression, insomnia, and weight gain.

Younger women usually begin menstruating again after chemotherapy, but women in or near their forties may not. For those who resume menstruating, fertility is not thought to be adversely affected.

Overall, chemotherapy has improved to the point where many women are able to continue working or keep up their normal routines during the treatment period. Side effects are milder and more manageable than they used to be. They are not insignificant, but they need not put your life completely on hold.

You might find it helpful to weigh the temporary unpleasantness of chemotherapy's side effects against the treatment's ability to destroy your cancer. Remember that chemotherapy, both with and without hormone-blocking therapy, increases survival rates. This may help you keep perspective as you deal with the effects of your treatments.

Note that many times, cancer patients misinterpret side effects of chemotherapy, such as fatigue and loss of appetite, as signs that their cancer is returning. Even though this may not be the case, discuss any such fears with your doctor.

7

Radiation Therapy

Radiation for cancer treatment is delivered to specified areas of the body in the form of a radiation beam, delivered by a machine called a *linear accelerator*. Its purpose is to destroy any undetectable cancer cells that might remain in the chest or breast after surgery and to reduce the possibility of a recurrence. Radiation is also sometimes used when cancer recurs, if the recurrence is small and localized. However, since radiation can be delivered to an area only once, a recurrence in a previously irradiated location will be treated only with surgery and adjuvant therapy.

How Radiation Works

Radiation destroys cells as they are reproducing, and it is most effective against rapidly dividing cancer cells. Radiation also damages healthy tissue, but the healthy tissue heals, and the cancer cells do not. Even so, it is important to target the cancer or the cancerous area as precisely as possible, minimizing the exposure of normal cells.

Radiation has been used in cancer treatment since the 1920s. Its risks used to be much higher than they are today. Damage to healthy organs was more widespread. New cancers, created by the radiation, were more common. As a result, you might feel nervous about radiation treatments. However, over the years, radiation therapy has grown more sophisticated. Modern equipment can produce electromagnetic radiation—a combination of X-rays and gamma rays—at higher energy levels than in the past. This allows radiation to be delivered more precisely to the targeted area, with less damage to normal cells. Usually, the radiation beam enters the body at an angle, passing through the cancerous area and out into the air, with minimal exposure of internal organs and healthy tissue.

Today, there is only a 1 percent risk that radiation treatments will cause a new cancer. For reasons that are not yet clear, the risk applies mainly to younger women. For women over forty, it is almost nonexistent.

Finding the Right Specialist

A *radiation oncologist* (an M.D. who specializes in radiation therapy) will likely be affiliated with a specialized radiation facility, which is usually part of a cancer treatment center or medical complex. Your surgeon might recommend that you meet with a radiation oncologist even before you have had your surgery. This does not automatically mean you will undergo radiation. It is an opportunity for the radiation oncologist to consult with you about the benefits and risks of treatment. This doctor will probably be someone your surgeon has worked with many

I had six weeks of radiation. I was so tired, sometimes I would just sit in a chair and sleep for an hour or more. I learned that it's okay to be tired, because your body is telling you it needs rest. After surgery and chemotherapy, I also had radiation. I got great support from family and friends. I kept telling myself I would beat this disease.

—Shirley, 58

times, and that may be sufficient to win your trust. If not, ask for another referral.

Consider taking a friend or your partner with you when you meet with the radiation oncologist for the first time or two, to help you remember the conversation. You might ask your companion to take notes. You will probably want to ask some or all of the following questions:

- How will radiation affect my chance of survival?
- How many treatments will I require, and how long will they take?
- How much healthy tissue will be exposed to radiation, and where?
- What side effects should I expect, and how can I manage them?

If you live in a rural area or small town, there may be no qualified radiation facility, and therefore no radiation oncologist, within several miles or more. Again, your surgeon will know where the nearest facility is located. Or you can call the Cancer Information Service (CIS) of the National Cancer Institute (NCI). See the Resources section in the back of this book.

If the nearest radiation facility is too far away for a daily commute, and if you are sure you want a lumpectomy with radiation, rather than a mastectomy (which probably would not require radiation afterward), you may need to make temporary living arrangements near a radiation facility during the weeks of your treatment.

When Is Radiation Used?

After Lumpectomy

Radiation therapy is recommended for most lumpectomy patients in order to destroy any random cancer cells that might remain in the breast or lymph nodes after surgery. Even when the entire tumor and a clean margin have been removed, along with affected lymph nodes (if any), it is still possible for a few undetected cancer cells to remain. Without radiation, cancer will reappear in the same area in about 30 percent of women. With radiation, the risk of recurrence drops to only 5 percent. The entire breast area is treated by radiation after lumpectomy, including the site from which the tumor was removed.

> *Breast cancer is like speed bumps in the road. You have rough days or rough procedures, but it gets better. You get over them.*
>
> *—Kristine, 51*

After Mastectomy

A full mastectomy is usually not followed by radiation because it is likely that all the cancer has been surgically removed. However, post-mastectomy radiation may be used if the tumor was large, or if cancer was found in several lymph nodes, and/or if cancer was found in the surgical margins (the edges of tissue left intact around the area where the tumor was removed). In such cases, radiation can be a safeguard in case the surgery did *not* remove all the cancer cells.

Similarly, if a good deal of cancer has been removed from the inner breast (near the breastbone) or has been found in several underarm nodes, radiation may be used on the lymph nodes behind the breastbone and above the collarbone, since these could contain cancer cells.

Finally, when a very large tumor (5 centimeters or more) has had to be shrunk by chemotherapy before surgery, radiation will be used after the surgery in an attempt to reduce the risk of local recurrence.

Treatment Planning

If you and your doctors determine that radiation is advisable for you, you will meet with your radiation oncologist to plan these treatments in detail. With the aid of a computer, the area to be treated will be pinpointed exactly and the amount of radiation calculated. The boundaries of the treatment area will then be marked either with indelible ink or with tiny tattoos, which will guide the technician who administers the treatment. Tattoos are permanent, but ink markings—even indelible ink—will eventually wash away.

The combination of being marked with tattoos or ink and then having to remain partially nude during radiation treatment can cause emotional discomfort. Knowing about these procedures in advance seems to help. Taking a friend or your partner with you for the first treatment or two might also ease your anxieties; however, your companion will not be allowed in the room with you during the actual treatment.

Undergoing Treatment

Radiation treatment sessions, including preparation time, may last about ten to twenty minutes. The radiation beam may be on from seconds to a few minutes each time. The treatments are usually given every weekday over a period averaging five to six weeks. Most women do not feel the radiation at all. A few report warmth, or a tingling sensation, but no pain.

Once treatments begin, you will soon become familiar with the routine. You will be asked ahead of time to avoid using any deodorants or per- fumes. Once at the treatment center, you will remove your clothes from the waist up and put on a gown. Then you will lie on your back, or perhaps on your side, with the radiation machine above you. Only a small segment of the entire area outlined by ink or tattoos will be treated at a time. Usually no more than two segments are treated each day, and the machine will be carefully positioned for each new segment.

You will need to lie still while each dose of radiation is given. Throughout the weeks of your treatment, you will be given occasional blood tests to make sure that the radiation is not affecting your blood count.

Radiation was not a bad experience. I actually came to enjoy going every day. In fact, I cried on my last visit because everyone there was so wonderful to me.

—Sandy, 44

Boost Treatments

After your initial five or six weeks of radiation therapy, you may immediately undergo an extra week or two of treatments that zero in on the site from which the tumor was removed. Whether you receive this "booster" dose of radiation will depend on the size of your tumor, the width of the margins taken from around the tumor, the size of your breast, and the kinds of equipment available to your radiation oncologist.

Sometimes boost treatments are delivered by the same kind of machine, a linear accelerator, but use a different kind of radiation beam—an *electron beam*. Electrons—small, radioactively charged particles—deliver radiation that does not penetrate as deeply as electromagnetic radiation. The treatment is therefore easier to confine to the targeted area and less likely to reach healthy tissue.

Studies show that boost treatments further reduce the risk of recurrence for all women but especially for those at greatest risk—women who are forty or younger. Younger women have longer life spans—more years in which they may have a recurrence; and, younger women are susceptible to more aggressive cancers.

Brachytherapy

Traditional radiation treatments are delivered by an external beam of radiation, aimed at a part of the body. Another technique, *brachytherapy*, delivers radiation from inside the body, to exactly the location where the treatment is needed. Brachytherapy has been successful in treating prostate cancer in men, and it is now being studied and used in a few medical centers for early-stage breast cancer.

Brachytherapy begins with the insertion of several tiny, flexible tubes (*catheters*) into the area from which the tumor was surgically removed. Catheters used for brachytherapy are also called *temporary radiation implants*. They remain in place throughout the five days of the treatment. Twice a day, the catheters are attached to a machine that delivers a high dose of radiation through the catheters directly to the area where the tumor was removed. The treatments last about ten minutes and are painless.

Brachytherapy has several advantages over traditional radiation. The main one is that the dose of radiation is tightly concentrated on the area of the breast from which the tumor was removed, so less radiation reaches the skin, inner organs,

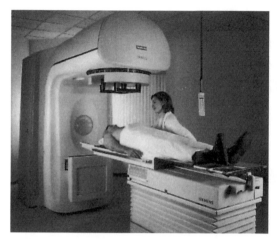

A patient receives an external-beam radiation treatment. *Photo courtesy of Sieman's Medical Systems, Inc.*

and healthy breast tissue. Brachytherapy also takes much less time than external radiation—a total of five days instead of five or six weeks. This is usually welcomed news to women with busy lives, and it can be especially important to women who live far away from the nearest radiation facility.

Brachytherapy has disadvantages as well. Because it is highly concentrated, it has only local effects and does not act against cancer cells that may be outside the treated area. It can also leave the skin somewhat firmer or darker in some women.

A form of brachytherapy is also used to deliver a boost treatment after a very small tumor has been removed. In this instance, the implanted catheters are filled with radioactive pellets, or seeds. The catheters are left in for three or four days, giving off the necessary booster dose. This usually requires a hospital stay to prevent the radiation from contaminating other people.

Side Effects

Radiation, like surgery, is a *local* treatment for cancer, meaning it mostly involves only the area in which cancer may be located. Temporary side effects from radiation treatment may include:

- swelling of the area
- redness resembling a sunburn
- fatigue
- soreness with swallowing (if the radiation beam is near the throat)

Long-term side effects may include:

- reduced skin elasticity
- a firmer-than-normal breast
- change in the size of the treated breast
- change in sensitivity to touch or pressure
- slight darkening or thickening of the skin

Radiation therapy does not adversely affect a woman's fertility, menstrual periods, or reproductive system. Some women are even able to breast-feed their babies with the untreated breast.

It is a good idea to take special care of yourself during radiation treatment. For example, you can minimize certain side effects, or just keep yourself more comfortable, by taking the following steps:

- Get plenty of rest.
- Use lukewarm water and mild soap to wash the treated area.
- Wear loose, comfortable clothing during the weeks of treatment, and if possible, avoid wearing a bra.
- Don't use powders, creams, lotions, or deodorants on the treated area before a treatment.

- Ask your radiation oncologist to recommend an aloe cream or vitamin cream to use on treated skin *after* treatments.
- Avoid exposing the treated area to the sun. Some physicians recommend wearing protective clothing or using sunscreen for up to one year following radiation treatment.
- Don't try to scrub or rub off any ink marks—they will fade in time. Tattoos, however, are permanent.

These measures, and any others that keep you comfortable, lift your spirits, or manage your side effects, can help you feel more in control—a good thing in a difficult time.

9

If Cancer Recurs

If your breast cancer has responded well to therapy, you have every reason to celebrate—treatments have worked, you have survived, and your life can return to normal. However, if you are like most women, somewhere in the back of your mind you fear that the cancer will recur or that a new cancer will develop in your other breast. You may also worry that your breast cancer has put your daughter, sister, mother, or granddaughter at higher risk.

Some women first confront these kinds of fears when the initial shock of diagnosis wears off and surgery is over. Others don't begin worrying until they have finished radiation therapy or adjuvant therapy. When you stop making frequent visits to familiar doctors and nurses, you may feel strangely vulnerable. For example, you may feel a wave of anxiety with every small headache or bodily pain, certain that the cancer is back.

Fortunately, the anxieties subside with time. Most women begin relaxing a little after each checkup until two years, and then five, have finally passed. Although breast cancer has been known to recur as late as twenty-five years after the first diagnosis, it is most likely to reappear within the first five years, and especially the first two. After the ten-year mark, a woman's risk of recurrence is very small.

Risk of Recurrence

Earlier, we discussed the general risks linked to primary breast cancer—the various environmental, hereditary, and behavioral factors thought to play a role in the development of this disease. To understand your risk of recurrence, consider these factors as well as the ones associated with your particular kind of breast cancer.

The same cancer characteristics that were used to guide your treatments will also help to estimate your risk of recurrence. These characteristics include:

- tumor size
- lymph node involvement
- presence or absence of hormone receptors
- whether the cancer cells are well differentiated, and thus do not divide very often, or poorly differentiated and divide frequently
- whether the cells are diploid (with normal amounts of DNA) or aneuploid (with abnormal amounts of DNA)
- the percentage of cells that are dividing in the tumor at any given time (the S-phase fraction)
- possibility of undetectable cancer cells remaining in your body

If breast cancer does reappear, it may do so at the site of the original tumor as a *local recurrence,* or in another part of the body as a *distant recurrence,* or *metastasis.* Although breast cancer may metastasize (spread) to many different locations, the most common (besides the lymph nodes) are the liver, lungs, brain, and bone. Bone is the most likely site for a recurrence. It seems to provide breast cancer cells with the kind of tissue and blood supply they need in order to thrive and multiply.

Ask your doctor about your specific risk of recurrence, but keep in mind that all risk factors, taken together, still amount to an indication, not a prediction. Most tumors possess a mixture of "good" and "bad" characteristics, making it difficult to say for sure how a cancer will behave. Living each day with hope and a positive attitude can go a long way toward redeeming a less-than-positive prognosis.

You can also increase your chance of long-term survival by paying close attention to your body. By now, you are very familiar with the signs and symptoms of breast cancer. Make sure you know the warning signs associated with a recurrence of breast cancer. Let your doctor know at once if you experience:

- bone pain
- headaches
- muscle weakness
- shortness of breath
- persistent cough
- weight loss or lack of appetite

Risk of a New Cancer

It is only fair to think that if you have had breast cancer once you should not have to worry about it twice. But cancer is never fair, and sometimes a new primary cancer does develop, in a breast treated with lumpectomy, in the untreated breast, or, less commonly, in a small amount of breast tissue left behind after mastectomy. Fortunately, the risk of a second breast cancer remains small—about 0.5 percent to 1 percent per year after your first diagnosis. If you have had a very aggressive cancer, you may be more likely to develop breast cancer again.

Follow-Up Care and Prevention

Your follow-up care will be more frequent and comprehensive during the first year or so after your surgery. Depending on your individual needs, you may visit your cancer surgeon, radiation oncologist, medical oncologist, and plastic surgeon (if you have had reconstruction). Your primary physician, the one who has coordinated your care throughout your treatment, will probably be involved in your follow-up care as well. He or she should be in touch with all the members of your medical team throughout the follow-up period, and you will probably see this doctor every six months or so for a complete physical examination. Your primary physician or other doctors may also order diagnostic tests as part of follow-up care.

> *I decided not to hide my breast cancer and told everyone I knew. I was astounded how many people gave me love, support, and prayers.*
>
> *—Marie, 45*

Blood Tests

After you have had chemotherapy, you will probably have monthly blood tests until your blood counts stabilize. Your doctor might also use blood tests that look for *tumor markers,* abnormally high amounts of certain body substances (such as certain kinds of proteins) that might indicate a tumor is present. The tests are not sensitive enough to find a recurrence at its earliest stages, since a tumor must be large enough to release detectable amounts of the marker substances. Results sometimes include false negatives. Thus the most appropriate use of these tests is in following a known recurrence to gauge its response to therapy.

Other blood tests look for elevated levels of enzymes that sometimes indicate the presence of cancer in the liver or bone. If test results suggest a problem with the liver, you will probably be given a CAT scan to investigate further. If tests show that bone cancer could be present, or if you experience bone pain, your doctor will order a bone scan.

Bone Scans

The first step in a bone scan is injection of a liquid containing low-level radioactive particles into the bloodstream. After a few hours, the particles are taken up by the bones, where they concentrate in areas of increased blood circulation. Such areas, called "hot spots," are detected by a machine that scans your body from above while you are lying on a table. However, hot spots can appear for many reasons—injury, arthritis, or other problems besides rapidly dividing cancer cells—and the machine cannot distinguish the cause. Therefore, if a bone scan finds an area of increased circulation, it will be followed up by an X-ray, CAT scan, or MRI, which show more clearly what is going on at that site.

Chest X-rays

Your doctor will also order a chest X-ray if you experience shortness of breath or develop a persistent cough.

BSE and Mammography

Of course, self-examinations and mammograms remain critical after cancer treatment. If you have had a lumpectomy, you should examine both breasts and the entire breast area. If you have had a mastectomy, you should examine your untreated breast, the surgical site, and the surrounding area, paying attention to your incision and chest wall for thickness, lumps, or rigidity. Report any suspicious changes immediately.

I offered as much emotional support to my mom as possible. I listened. I went with her to doctor appointments; I asked questions and took notes.

—Laura, 30, daughter

Most experts recommend a mammogram about six months after treatment. If you have had a lumpectomy, a mammogram of the surgically treated breast will serve as a new baseline. If you have had a mastectomy, a physical examination of your incision, armpit, breast area, and the area above your collarbone will be sufficient—but of course you should have routine mammograms done on your opposite breast. Some physicians recommend mammograms every six months for the first year or two after cancer treatment, then annually after that.

Hormone-Blocking Therapy

If your original tumor tested positive for hormone receptors, you have probably already begun a five-year course of hormone-blocking therapy, most likely with tamoxifen. This drug has been shown to prevent primary breast cancer in some high-risk women and has kept it from recurring in women who have already had breast cancer. Its effectiveness is clear, based on long-term research trials in which the incidence of cancer was reduced among the women taking tamoxifen. The drug also shrinks existing tumors and is used against breast cancer metastases. It kills cancer cells by preventing them from dividing. Like all anti-cancer drugs, it has risks and side effects as well as benefits, so you should ask your doctor to discuss these with you.

Guarding Against Cancer in Bones

The drug pamidronate (Aredia) belongs to a class of drugs called *bisphosphonates*, which disrupt the normal cycles in which bone breaks down and regenerates to keep the skeletal system healthy. Drugs in this class are used to treat osteoporosis, but studies show that they can sometimes prevent the spread of breast cancer to bone or treat the cancer if it does spread. Pamidronate is the most commonly prescribed bisphosphonate for this use. If your doctor thinks it would be beneficial in your case, you will probably receive an injection of pamidronate every few weeks.

Possible side effects of this drug are abdominal cramps, confusion, and muscle spasms; however these effects are less common when the drug is given in doses of 60 mg or less.

Treatment for Recurrence

Local Recurrence

Cancer that reappears at the site of the original tumor, in a breast that was treated with lumpectomy, is one form of local recurrence. It sometimes means that the cancer was not completely removed the first time, so technically, in these cases, it is not a true recurrence. In most cases of local recurrence in the treated breast, a mastectomy will be performed, both to make sure that all the cancer is removed and because radiation cannot be used a second time. Too much tissue damage is sustained if an area receives radiation more than once.

Local recurrence after mastectomy can appear in the surgical scar, in the skin or fat where the breast was, in the muscle or bone of the chest wall, or in a remnant of breast tissue left behind after the surgery. In this latter case, again, the cancer might be some of the original tumor rather than an actual recurrence. In any case, surgery is the first line of treatment, to remove the cancer and any affected tissue, muscle, or bone. If the original mastectomy has not have been followed by radiation, radiation can now be used on the entire breast area to eradicate any microscopic traces of the cancer.

Most cases of local recurrence are treated locally, with surgery and in some cases radiation. If the original tumor tested positive for hormone receptors, the woman will likely be on a five-year regimen of tamoxifen or other hormone blocker. But if there is a chance that the local recurrence signals a wider metas-

> *I always wonder if the cancer will return. I don't always talk about it, but the scare is there at times. One day at a time   that's how you live with cancer.*
>
> —*Liz, 42*

tasis, chemotherapy will be prescribed as well. For example, if the recurrence is in the mastectomy scar, the cancer has probably traveled there through the bloodstream and lymph nodes. The danger, of course, is that it has traveled elsewhere in the body as well. In this case, chemotherapy may stem any microscopic spread of the disease.

Metastasis or Distant Recurrence

When breast cancer has spread to another part of the body, treatment must be as aggressive as possible, while keeping side effects tolerable. The same therapies are available for metastases as for a primary cancer—surgery, radiation (in areas not previously irradiated), chemotherapy, and hormone-blocking therapy. However, the various treatments may be used differently, and in different combinations or sequences, than with a primary cancer. For example, if cancer has spread to an area where surgery is not advisable, radiation alone is sometimes successful both in relieving the pain of mestastasis and destroying the new tumor. In some other cases, if a new tumor is localized and readily accessible to surgery, the recurrent cancer can be removed. Adjuvant therapies may be needed in some cases.

Different chemotherapy drugs may be used in different combinations for breast cancer metastasis than for primary breast cancer. The focus among researchers is to develop new chemotherapy treatments that are at least as effective as ones currently in use, but with milder side effects and fewer risks.

Quality of Life

Whether your cancer recurs or you just worry that it will, there are any number of things you can do to boost your confidence, protect your well-being, and help you feel in control over important aspects of your life. Many breast cancer survivors suggest living one day at a time, paying attention to the things that matter most. These might include eating well, exercising, meditating, pursuing a spiritual search, finding creative expression, and nurturing the relationships that sustain you. Try to reestablish routines and challenges that were interrupted by your illness. Add new ones, ways of reaching out and enriching your life.

As discussed earlier, a support group can offer priceless help and new friendships. You might even consider working with organizations that promote breast cancer awareness and research. You might work with survivors like yourself or with women just recently diagnosed, who need to see what you represent—life going on. Activism has been responsible for many strides against breast cancer in recent years. You could make a difference by battling this disease on a new front, in small or energetic ways. There is always something you can do. Your life remains your own.

When my cancer recurred, I was really angry. I told my sister, 'I can't do it.' But she convinced me that I did it once and I could do it again.

—Jean, 48

In Good Company
(an inner dialogue)

"What do you mean, it was cancer?"
(I am too busy for that.)

"Yes, I'll be there in the morning."
(I don't mind losing a breast.)

"Please turn the morphine pump higher."
(Oh my God, this really hurts.)

"Your chemo will last only six months."
(Oh, well, a baby takes nine.)

"Is that a wig? You look stunning!"
(Surely he's flattering me.)

"Welcome: Breast Cancer Support Group."
(I am in good company.)

—*Suzanne W. Braddock, M.D.*

Resources

American Cancer Society (ACS)
15999 Clifton Rd NE
Atlanta, GA 30329-4251
Phone: 800-ACS-2345 (800-227-2345)
www.cancer.org

With more than 2 million volunteers and 3,400 local units, ACS works toward cancer treatment, prevention, and diminishing suffering through research, education, patient services, advocacy, and rehabilitation. The web site offers news and health information about the nature of breast cancer and its causes, risk factors, and latest treatment strategies. The site also features message boards and chat rooms.

Cancer Care, Inc.
275 7 Ave.
New York, NY 10001
Phone: 212-302-2400 (800-813-HOPE)
www.cancercare.org

A nonprofit organization since 1994, Cancer Care offers emotional support, information, and practical help to people with all types of cancer and their loves ones. All services are free. Forty-five oncology social workers are available for phone consultations in which they provide emotional counseling and support. Cancer Care also offers education seminars, teleconferences, and referrals to other services.

The Susan G. Komen Breast Cancer Foundation

5005 LBJ Freeway
Suite 250
Dallas, TX 75244
Phone: 972-855-1600
Fax: 972-855-1605
www.komen.org
www.breastcancerinfo.com

The Susan G. Komen Breast Cancer Foundation is a nonprofit organization with a network of volunteers working through local affiliates and *Race for the Cure* events in cities across the United States. Their mission is to eradicate breast cancer as a life-threatening disease by advancing research, education, screening, and treatment.

Y-Me National Breast Cancer Organization

212 W. Van Buren, Suite 500
Chicago, IL 60607
Phone: 312-986-8338
Fax: 312-294-8597
24-hour Y-ME National Breast Cancer Hotlines:
800-221-2141 English
800-986-9505 Spanish
www.Y-ME.org

The mission of the Y-ME National Breast Cancer Organization is to decrease the impact of breast cancer, increase breast cancer awareness, and to ensure through information, empowerment, and peer support that no woman faces breast cancer alone. Founded in 1978, Y-ME has matured from a kitchen-table support group of 12 women to a national organization with affiliate partners in 27 cities throughout the United States. The Web site is available in both English and Spanish versions.

National Coalition for Cancer Survivorship (NCCS)

1010 Wayne Avenue
Suite 770
Silver Spring, MD 20910-5600
Phone: 301-650-9127 or 877 NCCS-YES (877-622-7937)
Fax: 301-565-9670

Founded in 1986 by and for people with cancer and those who care for them, NCCS is a patient-led advocacy organization working on behalf of people with all types of cancer and their families. Their mission is to ensure quality cancer care for all Americans by leading and strengthening the survivorship movement, empowering cancer survivors, and advocating for policy issues that affect cancer survivors' quality of life.

National Cancer Institute
National Institutes of Health
Bethesda, MD 20892-2580
Phone: 301-496-4000
800-4-CANCER (800-422-6237)
Fax: 800-624-2511 or 301-402-5874
www.cancernet.nci.nih.gov

The NCI Web site offers recent cancer information from the National Cancer Institute, a component of the National Institutes of Health. Comprised of 25 separate institutes and centers, the NIH is one of 8 health agencies in the U.S. Department of Health and Human Services.

The Breast Cancer Fund
2107 O'Farrell Street
San Francisco, CA 94115
Phone: 415-346-8223
Fax: 415-346-2975
www.breastcancerfund.org

The Breast Cancer Fund (TBCF or The Fund) is a national nonprofit organization formed in 1992 to innovate and accelerate the response to the breast cancer crisis. The mission of The Fund is to end breast cancer and to make sure the best medical care, support services, and information are available to all women.

National Alliance of Breast Cancer Organizations (NABCO)
9 East 37th Street, 10th Floor
New York, NY 10016
Phone: 888 80-NABCO, or 888-806-2226
Fax: 212-689-1213
www.nabco.org

NABCO is one of the leading nonprofit information and education resources on breast cancer. A network of more than 400 member organizations nationwide, NABCO provides information to medical professionals and their organizations, and to patients and their families. It advocates beneficial regulatory change and legislation. With public and corporate partners, NABCO has collaborated on educational and medical programs that have reached a national audience, heightening public awareness and connecting women with needed services.

OncoLink

The University of Pennsylvania Medical Center
3400 Spruce Street – 2 Donner
Philadelphia, PA 19104
www.oncolink.upenn.edu/disease/breast

Maintained by the University of Pennsylvania, OncoLink's mission is to help cancer patients, families, health-care professionals, and the general public receive accurate cancer-related information at no charge. OncoLink offers comprehensive information about specific types of cancer, updates on cancer treatments, and news about research advances. The information (updated every day) is provided at various levels, from introductory to in-depth.

AMC Cancer Research Center & Foundation

1600 Pierce Street
Denver, CO 80214
Phone: 303-233-6501
800-321-1557
800-535-3777 Cancer Information and Counseling Line
www.amc.org

AMC Cancer Research Center is a not-for-profit research institute dedicated to the prevention of cancer and other chronic diseases. American Medical Center became the first institution in the country to devote its scientific resources entirely to the prevention of cancer. AMC is conducting cancer research in the areas of causation and prevention, nutrition in the prevention of disease, health communications, behavioral research, and community studies.

Blood and Bone Marrow Transplant (BMT) InfoNet

2900 Skokie Valley Road, Suite B
Highland Park, IL 60035
Phone: 847-433-3313
888-597-7674
Fax: 847-433-4599
www.bmtnews.org

BMT InfoNet is a nonprofit organization that provides information to bone marrow, peripheral blood stem cell, and cord blood transplant patients.

Celebrating Life Foundation (CLF)

P.O. Box 224076
Dallas, TX 75222-4076
Phone: 800-207-0992
www.celebratinglife.org

CLF is a nonprofit organization devoted to educating the African-American community and women of color about the risk of breast cancer. It also encourages advancements in the early detection and treatment, and the improvement of survival rates among these women.

The Avon Breast Cancer Crusade

www.avoncrusade.com

An initiative of Avon Products, Inc. that began in 1993, the mission of the Avon Crusade is to fund access to care and to find a cure for breast cancer. The organization puts a particular focus on medically underserved populations. The efforts of the Avon Crusade have made Avon the largest corporate supporter of the breast cancer cause. The Avon Crusade raises money to accomplish its mission in two ways: through the sale of unique "pink ribbon" fund-raising products, sold by more than 550,000 Avon independent sales representatives across the nation, and through the series of Avon Breast Cancer 3-Day events.

U.S National Library of Medicine
8600 Rockville Pike
Bethesda, MD 20894
www.nlm.nih.gov

MEDLINEplus
www.nlm.nih.gov/medlineplus

Produced by the National Library of Medicine, this site indexes articles from more than 3,500 medical journals. The service is aimed primarily at scientists and health professionals; however MEDLINEplus is written for consumers.

Healthfinder
www.healthfinder.gov

Healthfinder is a free guide to consumer health and human services information, developed by the U.S. Department of Health and Human Services. Healthfinder leads to on-line publications, clearinghouses, databases, Web sites, and support and self-help groups, as well as government agencies and not-for-profit organizations that produce information for the public.

National Lymphedema Network
Latham Square, 1611 Telegraph Ave. Suite 1111
Oakland, CA 94612
1-800-541-3259
www.lymphnet.org

This nonprofit organization provides education and guidance to lymphedema patients, health professionals, and the general public. Support groups are listed by state.

Glossary

A

adjuvant therapy: anticancer drugs used in chemotherapy and hormone blocking therapy, after surgery and/or radiation, to prevent recurrence or metastasis.

alkylators: a class of chemotherapy drugs that inhibit cell division and growth by replacing hydrogen in certain cell molecules.

anastrozole (*Arimidex*): a drug used in hormone-blocking therapy.

aneuploid: having abnormal amounts of DNA; tumors with aneuploid cells tend to be aggressive.

antibiotics: chemotherapy drugs that prevent the genetic material in cancer cells from reproducing.

antimetabolites: chemotherapy drugs that cause cells to die at the moment when they are ready to divide.

antimicrotubules: chemotherapy drugs that directly kill cancer cells with minimal damage to normal cells.

areola: the darker-colored skin surrounding the nipple.

aromatase: an enzyme that converts other hormones to estrogen; it is the principal source of estrogen after menopause.

aspiration: a procedure in which a hollow needle withdraws fluid from a breast mass or other part of the body.

asymmetrical: having opposite sides or parts that do not precisely match, as when one breast is larger or smaller than the other.

axilla: armpit.

axillary dissection: surgical removal of lymph nodes in the armpit area.

B

baseline: a condition against which later changes are compared, as in a *baseline* mammogram, usually taken before age forty.

benign: not cancerous.

bilateral: having two sides; affecting two sides equally, as in a *bilateral* mastectomy.

biopsy: a diagnostic procedure that removes tissue for microscopic analysis.

bone marrow: soft cell tissue in the bone center, where red blood cells, white blood cells, and platelets are manufactured.

bone marrow aspiration: the withdrawal of bone marrow to be analyzed for the presence of free-floating cancer cells.

bone scan: a diagnostic test that detects areas of increased blood circulation in the bone.

boost treatments: tightly focused, additional doses of radiation, usually given for a week or two after standard radiation treatments have ended.

brachytherapy: radiation treatments delivered to a precise location by a device implanted inside the body.

BRCA1, BRCA2: mutated genes associated with hereditary breast cancer.

breast implant: a soft pouch, filled with saline or silicone, that is surgically implanted beneath the skin and muscle of the chest wall to form a reconstructed breast after mastectomy.

breast reconstruction: any surgical method used to create a new breast after mastectomy. The new breast will not produce milk and will not have sensation but will look like a normal breast.

breast self-examination (BSE): a monthly routine in which a woman follows several steps to detect any changes or suspicious lumps in her breasts.

bulb: the smallest component in the milk-producing system of lobes in the breast.

C

cancer: a general term for diseases characterized by uncontrolled growth of abnormal cells that can invade and destroy healthy tissue. Also called malignancy.

carcinoma: the most common type of cancer, affecting skin, glands, or the lining of organs.

carcinogenic: cancer-causing.

CAT scan: a computer-aided method of creating three-dimensional images of organs and structures inside the body.

cell: the smallest structural unit of living tissue that can survive and reproduce on its own.

cell cycle: all cell activity from one cell division to the next.

chemotherapy: the administration of anticancer drugs that directly kill cancer cells or disrupt their ability to grow and reproduce.

clinical trial: a research project that tests drugs or other treatments on human subjects.

core biopsy: a diagnostic test in which a hollow needle removes small samples of tissue from a tumor for laboratory analysis.

cytologist: a specialist who analyzes cells and diagnoses disease from cell abnormalities.

cytotoxic: toxic to cells; capable of destroying cells.

cyst: a benign, fluid-filled lump.

D

DES (diethylstilbestrol): a synthetic estrogen that was once prescribed to prevent complications in pregnancy; it is no longer used, because it increases the risk of breast cancer.

DCIS (ductal carcinoma in situ): a pre-invasive cancerous condition in which abnormal cells have been found in the milk ducts of the breast but have not broken through the duct walls. DCIS will develop into invasive cancer if not treated.

diagnosis: the process of identifying a disease from its symptoms and from tests such as X-rays or biopsies; in breast cancer, determining the nature of a lump or any other change in the breast.

diagnostic mammogram: not a routine mammogram, but one ordered to investigate a lump found during BSE or a clinical examination.

digital mammography: a process in which the images produced on a mammogram machine are converted to computer code and then displayed in much finer detail than film can capture.

diploid: containing normal amounts of DNA; diploid tumors are usually not aggressive.

distant recurrence: a reappearance of cancer at a site other than the site of the original tumor.

DNA (deoxyribonucleic acid): the material that forms cells, carries the genetic code, and establishes hereditary patterns, including inherited risks for certain diseases.

duct: a narrow tube that carries milk from the lobes of the breast to the nipple.

ductal carcinoma: cancer that arises in the milk ducts.

ductal lavage: a diagnostic test in which a saline solution is introduced into the breast ducts and then withdrawn so that cells from the ducts can be analyzed for abnormalities.

E

early detection: discovery of a cancer while it is still small—no more than 2 centimeters in diameter—and before it has spread to lymph nodes near the breast.

enzyme: a complex protein that initiates certain chemical reactions in the body.

estrogen: a female sex hormone produced by the ovaries, adrenal glands, placenta, and fatty tissues.

estrogen receptor: a location on a tumor at which estrogen molecules can attach; the presence of estrogen receptors means tumor growth may be influenced by estrogen.

excisional biopsy: a surgical biopsy used for small tumors and capable of removing them completely.

exemestane (brand name Aromasin): a drug used in hormone-blocking therapy; it blocks estrogen production in postmenopausal women by inhibiting the enzyme aromatase.

expander: a soft, empty pouch placed behind the chest muscle and gradually filled with saline over a period of months to stretch the skin before a breast implant is put in place.

F

fibrocystic changes: a common condition in which the breasts develop benign, normal cysts that are sometimes mistaken for suspicious lumps. Often called fibrocystic disease, this condition is not actually an illness.

fine-needle aspiration (FNA): a kind of biopsy in which cells are withdrawn (aspirated) using a fine, hollow needle. In the case of breast cancer, the fluid is aspirated from a tumor, and the cells within the fluid are examined for evidence of cancer.

G

genetic: having to do with the genes and hereditary characteristics.

gluteal flap: a wedge of skin, muscle, and fat taken from the buttocks to be used in breast reconstruction.

H

hematoma: a mass of blood that collects in tissue or organs; breasts may be susceptible to hematomas after surgery.

hereditary: genetically passed on by a parent or parents to offspring; the risk for some cancers is hereditary.

hormone: a substance secreted by glands and circulated in the bloodstream to other parts of the body, where it exerts specific effects on cell activity.

hormone-blocking therapy: the use of drugs that block or disrupt the body's production of hormones in cases where a tumor depends on those hormones to grow.

hormone receptors: a location on a tumor at which either estrogen or progesterone molecules can attach; the presence of hormone receptors means tumor growth may be influenced by hormones.

hyperplasia: uncontrolled, abnormally fast growth of cells.

I

image-guided biopsy: a technique in which computer or ultrasound images are used to guide a biopsy needle to a lump that cannot be felt but has shown up on a mammogram; also called a stereotactic biopsy.

incisional biopsy: an open biopsy in which a small piece of a large tumor is removed for laboratory analysis.

inflammatory breast cancer: a particularly aggressive form of breast cancer usually treated with chemotherapy before surgery and radiation after surgery.

informed consent: a lengthy document that lists, for participants, all the potential risks, benefits, costs, and procedures of a clinical trial before it begins.

infusion: slow drip of medication directly into a vein.

in situ: a term meaning "in position" or "in its place"; a breast cancer that has not spread through the wall of the milk duct or lobe where it originated is called in situ.

invasive: cancer that is capable of invading, or has invaded, breast tissue beyond the wall of the duct or lobe in which it has arisen. Ductal carcinoma in situ (DCIS), if untreated, will eventually become invasive cancer. Lobular carcinoma in situ (LCIS) does not itself become invasive cancer but indicates a heightened risk.

L

latissimus dorsi flap: a section of muscle, skin, and some fat taken from the latissimus dorsi muscle of the upper back and used to form a new breast after mastectomy.

LCIS (lobular carcinoma in situ): the presence of abnormal cells within a lobe or lobes of one or both breasts; the cells have not spread beyond the walls of any lobes. The presence of LCIS indicates a heightened risk for either invasive lobular or ductal cancer.

letrazole (trade name Femara): a drug used in hormone blocking therapy; it blocks estrogen production in postmenopausal women by inhibiting the enzyme aromatase.

linear accelerator: the machine most commonly used to deliver radiation treatments.

lobe: one of fifteen to twenty rounded divisions in each breast; the part of the breast in which milk is produced.

lobule: one of several small components of a lobe.

local recurrence: reappearance of cancer at the site of the original tumor.

local treatment: treatment of cancer at the site of the tumor by surgery and/or radiation.

lumpectomy: breast cancer surgery that removes only the tumor and a surrounding margin of healthy tissue to be examined for cancer cells; also called a wide excision or partial mastectomy.

lymph, lymphatic fluid: a clear, yellowish fluid containing white blood cells that bathes body tissues and carries waste products away through lymph vessels.

lymph nodes: small masses of lymphatic tissue distributed along the lymph vessels and containing lymphocytes that filter waste products from lymphatic fluid.

lymph vessels: similar to blood vessels but with the purpose of circulating lymphatic fluid through the body and to the lymph nodes.

lymphedema: a persistent swelling in the arm caused by excess fluid that may collect when the lymph nodes and vessels are removed. This condition can occur at any time after surgery, including years later.

M

malignant: cancerous.

mammography: the use of X-rays to examine the breasts for tumors or microcalcifications.

mammogram: an image of the breast created by mammography.

margin: a ring of healthy tissue surrounding a tumor and removed at the same time as the tumor for laboratory analysis.

mastectomy: surgical removal of the breast.

mastitis: infection of the breast.

menopause: the permanent cessation of menstrual periods, usually in a woman's late forties to early fifties.

metastasis: the spread of cancer from its original site to another part of the body, usually through the bloodstream.

metastasizing: spreading to other parts of the body.

microcalcifications: tiny, grain-sized deposits of calcium in breast tissue, detectable by mammogram; when they appear in clusters, they may be a sign of DCIS.

micrometastasis: the early spread of cancer from the original tumor by means of random, microscopic cancer cells that have not yet formed a mass and are generally not detectable. (However, bone marrow aspiration can detect micrometastases when the cancer has begun to spread to bone.)

modified radical mastectomy: surgery that removes the entire breast and the axillary lymph nodes.

MRI (magnetic resonance imaging): a diagnostic imaging test that uses a powerful magnet and radio waves to show differences in the number of blood vessels in various types of body tissue. Cancerous tissue tends to have more blood vessels than healthy tissue.

multifocal: having more than one location; a multifocal breast cancer is present simultaneously in more than one lobe or duct.

mutation: a change in a cell's DNA.

myocutaneous: comprising muscle, skin, and fat; a myocutaneous flap is taken from one part of the body to reconstruct another, such as a surgically removed breast.

N

negative biopsy: one in which no cancer cells are seen in the tissue or fluid removed.

neoadjuvant therapy: chemotherapy or hormone-blocking therapy given before surgery to shrink a tumor to operable size.

node-negative: showing no evidence of cancer in the lymph nodes. A breast tumor is deemed node-negative when axillary dissection or sentinel node biopsy finds no cancer cells.

O

oncologist: a medical doctor who specializes in cancer treatment.

oncogene: a mutated gene associated with a heightened risk of cancer.

open biopsy: any surgical biopsy.

osteoporosis: a disease in which the bones become more porous and more susceptible to breakage as a person ages.

P

Pamidronate: one of a class of drugs called *bisphosphonates*, which have been shown in some studies to prevent the spread of breast cancer to bone or to treat the cancer effectively if it does spread.

partial mastectomy: surgery that removes only the part of the breast in which a tumor is located.

pathologist: a medical specialist who analyzes biopsied tissue under a microscope and diagnoses disease from any abnormalities that are present.

pathology report: the pathologist's written record of the analysis of biopsied tissue.

peau d'orange: skin texture like that of an orange; a symptom of inflammatory breast cancer.

pectoralis minor: a small, strap-like muscle running from the outer edge of the collarbone to the top of the breast, sometimes removed during axillary dissection.

PET (positron emission tomography): a diagnostic imaging test that reveals cell activity by detecting the different rates at which different cells consume sugar, or *glucose*. Cancer cells consume glucose more rapidly than normal cells.

phantom breast: the sensation that a surgically removed breast is still present.

plastic surgeon: a specialist in cosmetic and reconstructive surgery.

platelets: blood cells that aid clotting.

polygenic breast cancer: cancer that usually shows up in more than one member of an extended family.

port: a small, semi-permanent opening that is surgically implanted just under the skin. It is attached to a tube leading directly to a large vein. A port may be used when repeated injections are necessary, since it eliminates the need to tap a new vein each time.

postmenopausal: after menopause.

premenopausal: before menopause.

progesterone: a female sex hormone produced by the ovaries.

prognosis: the likely outcome of a disease; in the case of breast cancer, the statistical chance of long-term, disease-free survival.

prophylactic: preventive; a prophylactic mastectomy is performed when no cancer is present but the risk of breast cancer is high.

prosthesis: an external breast form worn by some women after mastectomy.

protocol: a document listing all steps, procedures, safety measures, and research methods to be used in a clinical trial.

Q

quadrantectomy: a partial mastectomy involving removal of the quadrant of the breast in which the tumor is located.

R

radical mastectomy: an invasive surgical procedure that removes the breast, the axillary lymph nodes, and the muscle of the chest wall; radical mastectomy is almost never used today.

radiation oncologist: a medical doctor who specializes in radiation therapy.

radiation therapy: a local treatment in which a radioactive beam is used to kill cancer cells in the area of the tumor.

radiologist: a medical doctor who specializes in the interpretation of X-ray images for diagnosis.

raloxifene: one of the class of drugs called SERMs, used in hormone-blocking therapy.

reconstructive surgery: the use of plastic surgery to model a new breast after mastectomy, using either breast implants or tissue from elsewhere in the body. The reconstructed breast looks like a normal breast but is not functional and does not have sensation.

recurrence: the reappearance of cancer after an initial course of treatment has ended; recurrence can be local or distant.

retraction: a drawing-in or drawing-back; when the nipple or the skin of the breast retracts, it can be a sign of inflammatory breast cancer.

S

S-phase fraction: the percentage of cells that are dividing in the tumor at any given time.

saline: a sterile, salt-water solution.

screening mammogram: a routine mammogram usually performed annually to check for indications of breast cancer.

sentinel node: the first lymph node to which lymphatic fluid drains from the area of a tumor; therefore, the first in which spreading cancer cells are likely to show up.

sentinel node biopsy: a procedure that removes the sentinel node for examination under a microscope. If the sentinel node is free of cancer, the other nodes do not need to be removed and examined, and surgery is minimized.

SERM (Selective Estrogen Receptor Modulator): one of a category of drugs that block either hormone production in the body or the hormone receptors on tumors, thus depriving certain cancers of the hormones they need for growth.

side effect: an undesirable effect of surgery, chemotherapy, radiation, or other treatment; some side effects include pain, nausea, skin changes, hair loss, or fatigue.

silicone: a synthetic material used to encase and fill some breast implants.

simple mastectomy: the surgical removal of all breast tissue but no lymph nodes; also called total mastectomy.

spiculated: star-shaped; a spiculated mass on a mammogram should be biopsied for cancer cells.

sporadic breast cancer: breast cancer in a patient with no known family history of the disease.

stem cell transplant: a procedure for regenerating bone marrow destroyed by high doses of chemotherapy drugs. Bone marrow stem cells (cells capable of forming blood cells), are removed before chemotherapy and then reintroduced afterward to restore bone marrow and its production of blood cells.

stereotactic biopsy: a technique in which computer images are used to guide a biopsy needle to a lump that cannot be felt but has shown up on a mammogram; also called image-guided biopsy.

systemic treatment: a cancer treatment such as chemotherapy that travels throughout the body to destroy random, microscopic cancer cells that may have spread beyond the site of the original tumor.

T

tamoxifen: an estrogen-blocking drug used in treating and preventing breast cancer.

taxane: one of several chemotherapy drugs (also called microtubules) that directly kill cancer cells with minimal damage to healthy cells.

tissue expansion: a process in which a soft, empty pouch is placed behind the chest muscle and gradually filled with saline over a period of months; this stretches the skin to accommodate a breast implant.

total mastectomy: the surgical removal of all breast tissue but no lymph nodes; also called simple mastectomy.

toxic: poison-like.

TRAM flap: a section of muscle, skin, and fat moved up from the lower abdomen to the chest area and used for breast reconstruction after mastectomy.

tumor: an abnormal growth of cells or tissue. Tumors can be benign (noncancerous) or malignant (cancerous).

U

ultrasonography: the use of high-frequency sound waves to generate images of internal organs or tumors. Ultrasonography can determine whether a suspicious lump is filled with fluid or is solid; if it is solid, it could be cancerous and should be tested further.

W

wide excision: removal of a breast tumor and surrounding margin of normal tissue; also called a lumpectomy.

Index

lump in breast, 5, 13
lumpectomy, 50–51
lymph, 2
    axillary nodes, 54
    excessive fluid, 59–61
    node sampling, 55
    nodes, 2, 5, 27–28
    presence of cancer cells,
    25
    vessels, 2
lymphedema, 56, 59–61

M

magnetic resonance imaging
    (MRI), 21–22
mammogram, 18–20
    diagnostic, 18
    digital, 18
    screening, 18
mammography, 18–20, 107
manual lymph drainage
    (MLD), 60
massage therapist, 60
mastectomy, 50–56
modified radical, 52–54
    partial, 50–51
    radical, 54
    simple, 52
    total, 52
mastitis, 7, 10
    see also breast infection
medical oncologist, 48, 78
meditation, 37–38
memory loss, 90

menopause, 90–91
metastasis, 4, 28, 103, 110
microcalcifications, 4, 20
micrometastasis, 56, 77
milk production, 2–3
modified radical
    mastectomy, 52–54

N

National Alliance of Breast
    Cancer Organizations
    (NABCO), 48
National Cancer Institute
    (NCI), 48, 94
National Cancer Society, 48
National Coalition for
    Cancer Survivorship
    (NCCS), 36
nausea, 88
neoadjuvant therapy, 80
nipple, 2–3
    discharge, 5, 16
    reconstruction, 74–75
    scaling, 16
    soreness, 16
nodes
    see lymph nodes
nutrition, 37–38

O

open biopsy, 23-25

P

pathologist, 24
peau d'orange, 7, 13

About the Authors

Suzanne W. Braddock, M.D., a breast cancer survivor, is a dermatologist in private practice in Omaha, Nebraska. Born and raised in New Jersey, Dr. Braddock received her medical training at the Medical College of Pennsylvania, Philadelphia, and at the University of Nebraska School of Medicine, Omaha. Dr. Braddock is the author of several scientific publications.

John Edney, M.D., F.A.C.S., a plastic surgeon in private practice in Omaha, Nebraska, specializes in post-mastectomy breast reconstruction and cosmetic surgery. Dr. Edney is an assistant clinical professor of surgery at the University of Nebraska School of Medicine, Omaha. He attended Creighton University School of Medicine. Dr. Edney and his wife, Pat, have three children—Christopher, Matthew, and Jennifer.

Jane Kercher, M.D., F.A.C.S., is a general and oncological surgeon in Denver, Colorado. She received her medical training at the University of Utah Medical School, Salt Lake City, and at the University of

Nebraska, Omaha. A native of Wyoming, Dr. Kercher now lives in Denver with her son, Matthew.

Melanie Morrissey Clark has worked as a writer and editor for more than fifteen years. She is editor in chief of *Today's Omaha Woman* magazine in Omaha, Nebraska, and is also co-author of *The Fertility Handbook—A Guide to Getting Pregnant* (Addicus Books, 2002). Ms. Clark is vice president of Clark Creative Group in Omaha. She holds a bachelor of science degree in journalism from the University of Nebraska. She lives in Omaha with her husband, Fred Clark, and their triplets—Cooper, Sophie, and Simon, born in 1997.

Addicus Books Health Titles

www.AddicusBooks.com

Please send:

_____ copies of _____

(*Title of book*)

at $ _____ each   TOTAL: _____

Nebr. residents add 5% sales tax   _____

Shipping/Handling
   $4.00 for first book.
   $1.10 for each additional book   _____

   TOTAL ENCLOSED: _____

Name _____

Address _____

City _____ State _____ Zip _____

❑ **Visa** ❑ **MasterCard** ❑ **American Express**

Credit card number _____ Expiration date _____

Order by credit card, personal check or money order. Send to:

Addicus Books
Mail Order Dept.
P.O. Box 45327
Omaha, NE 68145
Or, order **TOLL FREE: 800-352-2873**
or online at
www.AddicusBooks.com